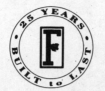

How Healthy Is Your Family Tree?

A Complete Guide
to Tracing Your Family's Medical
and Behavioral Tree

CAROL KRAUSE

Foreword by Leo Lagasse, M.D.

A FIRESIDE BOOK
Published by Simon & Schuster

New York   London   Toronto   Sydney   Tokyo   Singapore

For my sister Kathy

FIRESIDE
Rockefeller Center
1230 Avenue of the Americas
New York, NY 10020

FIRESIDE and colophon are registered trademarks
of Simon & Schuster Inc.

Manufactured in the United States of America

1 3 5 7 9 10 8 6 4 2

Library of Congress Cataloging-in-Publication Data
Krause, Carol.
How healthy is your family tree?: a complete guide to tracing your family's
medical and behavioral history/by Carol Krause.—1st Fireside ed.
      p.   cm.
1. Medical genetics. 2. Genealogy. I. Title.
            RB155.K69 1994
  616'.042—dc20   93–10187
                  CIP

CONTENTS

ACKNOWLEDGMENTS

My sincerest appreciation goes to Larry Mauksch of the department of medicine at the University of Washington Department of Family Medicine in Seattle. Our genogram model was genuinely a collaborative effort. It was eye-opening, a breakthrough, and fun. Thanks go also to Dr. Henry Lynch and Jennifer Cavalieri of the Hereditary Cancer Institute at Creighton University in Omaha. Their pioneering research gave me the foundation for this book, and has saved lives, including mine. On the subject of saving lives, I am grateful to Dr. Moshe Shike of the Memorial Sloan-Kettering Cancer Center (we must stop meeting that way).

To Dr. Leo Lagasse and Dr. Beth Karlan of Cedars Sinai Medical Center: Thanks for always answering my phone calls. I would like to offer special gratitude to Pam Perry and the Krannert Institute of Cardiology at the Indiana University Medical Center for overwhelming support on this project.

I want to thank the special people and families who shared their stories and secrets: Joyce Bates Campbell, heart patients Cindy Leffew and Harold Board, Tricia, and Danielle.

This work could not have been completed without the encouragement of several others in my personal world, especially Gail, Andre, Linda, and of course my friends at the Memorial Sloan-Kettering Post Treatment Center, including Vicki, Virginia, Irma, and all the others who showed me how to have spirit and strength.

Heartfelt appreciation to Robin Burke and Catherine Campbell for their research and friendship when I needed it the most. I must also thank Al Berman and Aviva Bobb for their help with research, and Stefan for his nimble fingers. My love and gratitude to Rebecca Schwaner, who graciously held down the fort on the West Coast, which freed me up to do my work.

Here's a special message for my friend Susan Silk: Thanks for understanding my absence during my year of writing and healing. And where would I be without my helper Chris Hippolyte, who keeps my head on straight, or Alexandra Penney, who believed I had something to say?

Because this is a list of acknowledgments, may the grandest nod go to my editor Mark Chimsky, who pursued my work and believed in this project, and who guided me through it with a calm and inquisitive eye.

The most loving thanks is reserved for my sisters Peggy and Kathy for their diligent genealogical work, to my sister Susan for showing us all how to have courage, and to my cousins, Barb, Judy, and Joanie for sharing the battle.

It is only appropriate that I remember my mother and father on this page, whose very distinctive genes live within me and continue their debate for my soul. And warmest thanks go to Zack, Emma, and Betsy for their unconditional love.

FOREWORD

*A*s we approach the twenty-first century we are seeing dramatic solutions to a host of previously unsolvable medical problems. Many of these advances are in genetics, a field which is destined to play a key role in the continuing medical revolution. Our inherited genetic tendencies are important predictors of our potential for genetic health and disease. Many people don't realize, for example, that it is a genetic alteration in individual cells that allows them to develop into cancer.

In this important book, *How Healthy Is Your Family Tree?*, we are presented with powerful reasons to increase our understanding of our own personal genetic inheritance. We are shown how to develop our own medical and behavioral family tree and thus uncover our unique inherited tendencies for common disorders such as heart disease or cancer or some other less common but sometimes serious conditions.

This exercise—a look at your family history—could change your life, freeing you from worry about health risks that are unlikely to occur while guiding you toward beneficial modification of life and behavioral patterns when the findings suggest it. If, for example, you discover a familial tendency toward heart disease, there are effective steps which could dramatically improve your potential to remain healthy. You could change to a low fat diet, increase your exercise or even take a cholesterol-lowering drug. Even though review of your family tree indicates a high risk, you might well avoid heart disease entirely with the proper steps.

What if you find a family tendency for cancer? Medical journalist Carol Krause points out that with appropriate screening and surveillance those cancers can often be prevented or detected at an early curable stage, as her personal case so vividly demonstrates.

Health conscious individuals wanting to increase their awareness of genetics and its effects on their future health will benefit in direct and important ways from this well-researched volume. Read it carefully with a pencil in your hand.

Leo Lagasse, M.D., Director,
Gynecologic Oncology, Cedars-Sinai Medical Center
and Professor of Obstetrics and Gynecology at
University of California at Los Angeles

INTRODUCTION

*T*his is your story. If you're anything like me, your life often feels like a hazardous excursion filled with sudden mishaps, interwoven with moments of joy.

In our struggle to understand why we do what we do, why we are what we are, and why things happen to us, it is tempting to look for that one-shot, instant-soup solution that will change the course of our lives.

Before you pick up that next self-help book, before you pay for a weekend seminar conducted by a commercially successful guru, consider this proposition: that the answers you seek may already exist in your most overlooked resource—within the tiny cells of your own body.

If you doubt this even for a minute, then please take the time to read my story and find out how knowing about my genetic past literally saved my life and gave me strength to face the newly resurrected time ahead of me. And then take the time to discover the clues within your own genes. Find out how the startling pace of medical research has opened up fresh opportunities for you to make remarkably realistic choices about your life and health.

I will show you how to look at your family tree in a new and exciting way. Once you've put your tree together, your life can suddenly make more sense. You will begin to believe that you are a part of a continuing plan and, like me, you may see that perhaps there truly is a method to the madness of our existence after all.

My Family's Story

"This is the saddest phone call I will ever make," my father said, preparing me for heartbreak. For months my mother had been having some vague "female" problems. Finally, her doctors decided she would have to have exploratory surgery. "It's cancer of the ovary," Dad said hoarsely. "The surgeon told me it looks like black rock salt sprinkled all over her lower half." My father's voice was trembling with a magnitude I never thought possible. "They say she has six months."

Mom was fifty-four years old. I was twenty-one. It was my first real experience with dreadful loss. After all, this wasn't supposed to happen until Mom was old, really old. The knowledge of her suffering and the anticipation of her death kept me awake at night, week after week.

She survived a year longer than predicted—a precious year that could have been spent looking back, but, instead, Mom urged us to look forward. She encouraged me not to cancel a planned European odyssey with a friend (youth-hostel-style). While I sent Mom postcards and ethnic dolls for her collection, my sister Kathy stuck close to home and began to work on a project that, ironically, would intervene with our own genetic destinies: She began to work on our medical family tree.

In all, there are four sisters in my family. Mom died in 1972, before the highly publicized death of comedienne Gilda Radner and the discoveries about the genetic links of ovarian cancer. But we knew we were somehow at risk. Kathy, with the help of my oldest sister Peggy, began to put together a rather ominous family tree. Cancer was cropping up all over its branches, but there were many different kinds of cancer, and we couldn't see any connection.

We quizzed my father, who said his sister Bertha had died of stomach cancer at the age of thirty-two. His own father, once a chef for the famous Pfister Hotel in Milwaukee, had died of colon cancer at age thirty-three. He showed us his father's death certificate and it was specific: cecal cancer. (The cecum is a little sac at the top of the colon.) At the time I didn't know how important that information would be. He had no death certificate for Bertha, and that, too, would become important.

Once Kathy compiled a sketchy medical family tree, she put it away for a while, and from time to time would hopscotch the country looking for more upbeat genealogical information. Over the next decade, she wrote to relatives who might have genealogical answers to questions about our family's midwestern history, but not much medical information surfaced.

My father eventually got remarried to a wonderful woman, and the rest of us went on to complete our educations and start careers. The fear of cancer was always there, like a tiny speck of dust in the eye that you can't rub away. But very little was known about cancer and genetics in the seventies and early eighties, and we were sure we wouldn't have to worry about it until we were at least our mother's age. So, for the next fifteen years, we continued our lives, blissfully ignorant of the horror that lay ahead.

My sister Peggy was twenty-seven when Mom died. Her first child, a boy, was born two months later. For us, his arrival was a joyous reaffirmation of the cycle of life. Over the next decade, Peggy would give birth to three more boys, each one a tender reminder of that joy.

Kathy finished law school and went on to become executive director of the Legal Aid

Foundation in Los Angeles, carrying with her Mom's legacy of compassion for others. Kathy's work became her passion, and she found herself too busy to marry. Instead, she spent much of her spare time updating the family's genealogy.

My youngest sister Susan received her Ph.D. in economics and became a government banking economist. Today she has a high-level job with the U.S. Comptroller of the Currency.

At the time of my mother's death, I went to Washington, D.C., to get a master's degree in communications and public affairs. I took my degree to a small television station in Evansville, Indiana, where I began a career in broadcasting. I met my husband Erik while working at the CBS station in Chicago and, in 1986, I gave birth to our son Zachary.

At seventy-one, Dad was being treated for cancer of the prostate, a not uncommon ailment at his age. But during treatment they made a troubling discovery: a separate primary tumor in the ureter. Thankfully, Dad's cancers were slow-growing, and for the first few years he was still active.

While Dad was in his final years, the news about Gilda Radner hit, and suddenly everyone was talking about ovarian cancer. Kathy dusted off the old family medical tree, and we felt compelled to update it. I asked Dad again about his sister Bertha. "Stomach or colon cancer," was all he could remember. It seems astonishing he would not remember how his sister died, but it was 1942, Bertha was newly married and lived far away, and my parents were preoccupied with my mother's mother, who was also dying of cancer. I made a mental note to try and find Bertha's death certificate.

We convinced ourselves that the cancer risk for us was too vague to prompt obsessive anxiety. By now our ages ranged from thirty-seven to forty-four, and we still thought we were too young to worry about it. Besides, the risk of ovarian tumors was greater when two close relatives were hit. Despite our grim medical family tree, only my mother had cancer of the ovary. We didn't yet realize that with new scientific research, even the limited information we had could be lifesaving.

In my Dad's final months there was some good news. Susan, at age thirty-seven, had fallen in love and was getting married. We knew it was likely to be the last big family event for my father, and I know he worked hard to hang on long enough to walk her down the aisle.

It was a poignant sight, seeing Dad walk Susan toward the altar, knowing that with each step he felt terrible pain. The cancer had invaded his spine, he was pale and shaky, but he walked with his body erect and his head held high, a proud father giving his beautiful daughter away in marriage.

Dad died a few months later, having lived through the cancer deaths of his father, sister, two brothers, and my mother. With each death, he had been the strong one for our extended family, the one who organized the medical care, the one who counseled the spouses, the children. When I said my silent good-byes at his deathbed, I wondered if I had inherited the strength I needed now.

Even then I saw my family medical history as more of a family curse, and not a scientifically explainable phenomenon. There were too many different kinds of cancer, from both sides of the family. And I assumed that very few cancers were thought to be genetic. I knew that breast cancer tended to run in families. But that was one of the few organ cancers we didn't have anywhere on our family tree. In fact, when it came to breast cancer, we seemed to have better odds than the average family. So I decided simply not to worry about it.

But my innocence was about to be shattered like a piece of delicate crystal slammed against a concrete wall. When my sister Susan was in town for Dad's funeral, she mentioned a mild but persistent pain in her side. She had been trying to get pregnant and was anxious to clear up any possible gynecological problems. A week later, her doctor determined she had an ovarian cyst. Susan told her doctors about my mother's medical history (ovarian cancer), but her gynecologist simply replied, "Oh, you're only thirty-eight, much too young to worry about that."

But the cyst seemed to get worse, and a couple of months later, her doctor decided it had to be surgically removed. What they found surprised everyone: a large cancerous tumor on the ovary, but, even worse, there was a separate cancer in her uterus that had already spread to a lymph node.

Kathy and I pored over our mother's medical records to find some answers. We viewed Susan's diagnosis as a clear sign that it was time to get serious and do some state-of-the-art analysis of our family history. Had Mom also had uterine cancer? Why would Susan have *two* cancers? What insidious combination of genes and circumstance would conspire to give Susan devastatingly serious cancers at the age of thirty-eight? For the first time, we knew for certain that our family tree was the key.

We got together as much information as we could and began to consult experts in oncology (the study of tumors) and medical genetics. We quickly learned that only a few doctors are truly competent in the genetics of cancer, and we did a lot of research to find the right ones. But the answers they gave us were hard to stomach. With a mother and a sister with ovarian cancer, the other three sisters were at serious risk. Each of us had a fifty-fifty chance of getting it, we were told. And sooner rather than later. We learned that inherited cancers usually hit one, two, even three decades earlier than sporadic cancers.

But that was only the beginning of the nightmare. The experts told us some other shocking news. It appeared our family had been hit by a *syndrome* of cancers. What? I had never heard of such a thing!

"Cancer of the colon, uterus, and ovary can be connected," we were told by Dr. Leo Lagasse at the Cedars-Sinai Cancer Center in Beverly Hills, California. "You must have your colons checked immediately, and consider having your uteruses and ovaries surgically removed."

I was in the midst of trying to have a second baby. At age forty-two, Kathy, a physically-fit jogger and health-food consumer, was hoping

she still had time to start a family. Peggy, at age forty-five, was finished having babies, but had difficulty accepting the notion that she should have healthy organs removed. Everywhere we went, we took our medical family tree with us, and everywhere the advice was the same: "Get those organs out and get them out fast."

We did not take this advice lightly. Removing the ovaries meant the loss of precious natural estrogen. This could result in early bone damage (osteoporosis), decades of medication, and symptoms of old age that might come years sooner for us than for women who go through the natural evolution of menopause.

Susan bravely began her chemotherapy and radiation treatments, while Peggy and Kathy scheduled their hysterectomies. I decided to wait a couple of months until I completed a move from Los Angeles to New York (and because I felt the only sane thing to do was for one of us to be off the medical merry-go-round—at least for the time being).

Before their surgeries, Peggy and Kathy each underwent a colonoscopy, a procedure in which a flexible tube is threaded into the intestines. Their colons looked normal, and we wondered if such an invasive procedure had been necessary. Their doctors had also insisted on mammograms, because breast cancer can sometimes be part of the ovarian syndrome. There, too, they had a clean bill of health.

But Kathy's surgery resulted in another shocker. Dr. Lagasse found a tiny tumor in her ovary and an early malignancy in her uterus. At first they thought the cancers were caught early enough, but several months later, tiny ovarian tumors reappeared in the lining of her pelvis, even though the ovaries themselves had been removed. We were convinced she was genetically programmed for this disease and there was nothing she could have done to prevent it. But she now had a fighting chance only because doctors had our medical family tree and convinced her to act quickly.

I was happy to learn that Peggy, who was recuperating in the hospital room next to

Kathy's, was found to be cancer-free. Did the surgery save her life? We don't have any firm answers, but geneticists who later studied her ovarian tissues suspect that Peggy also had inherited a number of potentially deadly genes.

I was now looking at a mother and two sisters with ovarian cancer. How the uterine cancer fit in we weren't sure, but a glance at our medical family tree reminded us that our mother's mother, named Bird, was killed by a uterine tumor when she was sixty-two. To a medical geneticist, that is not an alarmingly early age, but when I sent for my grandmother's death certificate, it revealed the cancer had first struck when she was only fifty-six. Had Bird's genes combined with my mother's to form a deadly genetic cocktail?

No matter how I looked at it, my own risk was extraordinarily high. I had to get my ovaries and uterus removed. I was forty years old and was facing a forced early menopause. I would not be able to have any more children. But I desperately wanted to see my son Zachary reach adulthood, and that had to be my first priority. I scheduled the surgery, praying they would not find malignancies in my reproductive organs.

That's when my personal genetic map took a bizarre turn. My ovaries and uterus were cancer-free, but during the colonoscopy, doctors found a malignant tumor in my colon. In fact, it sat right in the cecum, the exact resting place of the tumor that killed my paternal grandfather, Ernst, when he was only thirty-three. It was an unwelcome genetic snake that slithered down the branches of my family tree. Twenty-five percent of my genes came from a grandfather I never knew—a deadly genetic bequest.

Another fact nagged at us. It even looked as if we had been programmed to get cancer at the same time, within six months of one other. We asked our doctors what would have happened if we had not done our medical family tree. It is likely that Kathy's cancers would have begun spreading through her body with reckless abandon, not showing symptoms for months. My colon tumor might not have shown symptoms for another year or so, and my chances would have been far worse. I did have to experience a difficult surgery, but I was spared chemotherapy. My tumor was discovered early *only* because we found aggressive, savvy doctors. Or, as a good friend pointed out, because we were aware enough to look for answers.

"Enough already," you're saying, but sadly my family's story is still evolving. When I was in the midst of writing this book, I received another phone call, from my sister Kathy, who was in the hospital, still undergoing treatments for her ovarian cancer. She told me that my cousin Joanie had had surgery for ovarian and endometrial cancer, and that they had removed a tumor the size of a grapefruit from her ovary.

I slowly sunk into my desk chair upon hearing this news. My cousin Joanie was forty-nine, and had been the healthy one in her family. She was now a dues-paying member of the Krause Cancer Club.

Two years before I had advised Joanie to get regular exams. "I meant to," she tells me now, "but things kept getting in the way." By the time she made her doctor's appointment, she was already feeling symptoms. Happily, her doctors took one look at her well-documented family history and acted aggressively, and Joanie has a good prognosis.

Joanie's disease was hauntingly similar to that which struck both of my sisters. It was another compelling reason for me to continue my vigilance for my own care. Just weeks before publication of this book, I waltzed into my radiologist's office for my annual mammogram (right on schedule) and came out with an unexpected jolt: a suspicious spot on my left breast that wasn't there a year ago. A biopsy revealed a very early malignancy. Surgery was quick, chemotherapy was not needed, and my prognosis is excellent. Another cancer caught early because I respected the information on my family tree, and took it seriously.

My sisters and cousins know it is our medical family tree that has given us all a chance to live.

BURIED SECRETS OF THE PAST

While not all families have stories as sobering as mine, all families do have a past. And family history can offer answers to the most mystifying questions—not just about health but about why we look and act the way we do.

Take, for example, the tale about the dwarf. A friend of mine tells a story about a woman who not long ago gave birth to a dwarf. I'm not sure what type of dwarfism the baby had, but the woman was told it was genetic—that she and her husband both carried a rare gene that combined to make such a special infant.

"That can't be," the woman told her doctor. "There is no instance of this anywhere in either family." When a genetic specialist confirmed the diagnosis, she set out to prove them wrong. What began as a simple family tree soon grew addictive. The woman became so fascinated with the people and stories on her side of the family that she became quite a skilled genealogist. Because her family had some minor royalty back in England, she was able to trace them back to the eighteenth century.

That's when she found him. A great-great-great-great-great grandfather actually served as a court jester at an important royal palace. The reason he had such a post, although he was a nobleman himself: He was of dwarfish stature.

The story makes an undeniable point: We all carry within us a mosaic of our biological past. Sometimes the pieces are ones we would prefer not to possess, but they are there, from conception to death. If we have children, some of these fragments are given new life, to potentially be passed on again and again.

The tale of the dwarf demonstrates that external physical characteristics are passed on through time. We all know that when we see a woman pushing a stroller carrying a baby that could be her clone.

But the scientific world is now paying more attention to the less obvious internal physical and behavioral secrets we have inherited from our ancestors that can cause good health, illnesses, and personality traits.

Certainly, there is still much debate over which shapes us more, our genes or how we were raised. But a look at your family history can be revealing and helpful in ways you might not have imagined.

Take the example of another friend who learned that you don't have to take your family tree back three centuries to get some answers. Max (that's what I'll call him) is struggling with a compulsive gambling problem. It wasn't until he lost most of his money and his wife threatened to leave him that he decided he'd better figure out why he, a law school graduate from a prestigious university and family, couldn't kick such a terrible habit.

First, he had several intense talks with his brother, who had undergone treatment for the same problem. Then he examined his relationship with his father and realized that his dad's frequent escapes to the racetrack to bet on horses were more than just a hobby. Max started to ask questions about his paternal grandparents, and made an intriguing discovery. They were apparently affluent, and had a strange unwritten pact that kept their marriage together. Every day his grandfather sent a car around to pick up his grandmother, who enjoyed betting at a nearby racetrack. His grandmother was given an allowance for this "recreation," which was fully spent each day.

A brother, father, and grandmother. All "sophisticated" gamblers. Was this the result of genes or environment? To Max it didn't much matter. Knowing that compulsive gambling runs in his family lifted the tonnage of guilt that had burdened his soul. "Maybe it's not totally my fault," he told me. His perfectionist ego now feels less assaulted, and he is able to focus more clearly on his therapy, rehabilitation, and protecting his son from the same fate.

Then there's my cousin Derby. Certainly there was no one more charming than Derby. He was a decade older than the kids in my immediate family, and at family get-togethers we would gather around him and giggle at his jokes and antics. I should point out that I come from a pretty straitlaced extended clan: a lot of church-goers with solid family ties and a genuine sense of what is right and wrong.

Derby eventually went into the travel business, but seemed to drift from job to job. Then one day some people complained that he had arranged a tour, taken their money, but that they never got their trip. Soon the IRS was after him, and he ended up spending some time in jail.

After jail, Derby continued to get great jobs, usually in public relations for hotels or travel agencies. Yet he never stayed in one position for very long, and we were mystified. Was he constantly being fired or was he simply restless? With his charm and clever tongue, he could always talk his way into a new situation. His last job was as a manager for a stock car driver in northern California. One day they took a small plane headed for a race somewhere, and the plane disappeared. While searchers looked for them, I had a long talk with my dad about my cousin.

"Derby was raised in a sane and normal home, wasn't he?" I asked. "His parents were not fast-talkers and would never get involved in scams or schemes, and neither would his sisters. Where did Derby get that urge to drift?"

"That's easy," Dad told me. "Derby's grandfather on his mother's side. Used to leave home for long periods of time and travel with a carnival, running God knows what kind of cons and scams."

A few days later they found Derby's plane in pieces, hidden by trees on a mountain ridge. With it crashed all of Derby's insatiable hopes and dreams. Will his death end the cycle of mischief that may have been locked in his genes? We may soon find out. Derby left behind three attractive and high-spirited children.

I

HOW YOUR GENES WORK

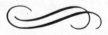

Study the past if you would divine the future.
CONFUCIUS

GENETIC GIFTS: HOW THEY ARE PASSED TO US

Scientists still don't know exactly which genes are passed to our offspring, but they do have some idea about how the gene pool will split. This I learned at a young age.

Amid the smell of formaldehyde and fertilizer, I was the subject of much scrutiny in my high school biology class. Of the four children in my family, I was the only one with blond hair, blue eyes, fair skin, and a number of other "recessive" genes. (For example, I can't curl my tongue, a deficit that embarrasses my seven-year-old son, who has inherited the all-important tongue-curling gene.)

None of this is anything to brag about, of course, but it started a debate among those who knew my dark-haired sisters. Was my hair a dye job? (They knew my light eyes were real, as these were pre–contact lens days.) My teacher let the insults fly for a while but then cleverly spun the conversation into a lecture on Mendelian genetics.

Peas and Presumably People

Gregor Mendel was an Austrian monk and botanist who lived in the nineteenth century. By mixing and crossing simple garden pea plants, he discovered some basic laws of genetics: that peas (and presumably people) inherit certain traits according to an average ratio.

How many genes do we carry in our body? How many traits could there possibly be? One hundred, a thousand, ten thousand? Get ready for an astonishing answer: The human body contains at least fifty thousand and possibly as many as one hundred thousand genes! Each one controls a trait of some sort—height, weight, hair color, blood type, intelligence, and so on.

You're Not Just One in a Million

The possibilities are staggering. We get half our genes from our father, half from our mother. The resting place for these genes is in our chromosomes. Sperm and ovum each have twenty-three chromosomes. Passed on with all of these chromosomes are the genes they contain.

A man can make up to 8 million genetically different sperm. A healthy man releases 140 to 400 million sperm during each act of sex, so many of the genes will be identical.

A woman also has the potential to produce 8 million genetically different ova, so in theory, a mom and dad have the capacity to produce 64 million genetically different offspring!

In reality, a woman produces only two hundred thousand to four hundred thousand ova in a lifetime, only a few hundred actually ripen in the ovaries, and only a handful of those ever get fertilized. As babies, we are handed a potpourri that is nothing short of a miracle for surviving the odds.

Mendel's Laws of Inheritance

In his garden laboratory, Mendel crossed a pea plant with yellow seeds with a pea plant with green seeds. The by-product: two *yellow*-seeded plants. From this, Mendel developed the idea that certain genes (he called them *factors*) are dominant—in this case, the yellow seeds. The ingenious monk then crossed his two hybrid yellow-seeded plants. To his surprise, of the four offspring, three were yellow but one turned up *green*.

These experiments led to three basic laws of genetics:

1. Genes come in pairs, one from your mother and one from your father.
2. Genes can mix, but they do not get diluted. Each single gene stays pure from generation to generation and could reappear at any time.
3. Each gene carries codes called *alleles*. Certain alleles are dominant, certain others are recessive. In other words, dominant genes can mask the presence of the recessive genes. This is why Mendel's first generation of pea plants had no green seeds, even though the green-seeded genes were passed down.

Mendel's Pea Plant Experiment

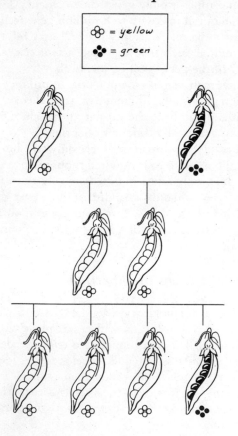

Here's how all of this works with one of the simple traits—eye color.

The genes controlling eye color consist of primarily two alleles: brown and blue. Brown is dominant, blue is recessive. You need two blue alleles to produce a blue-eyed baby. Here are the likely combinations:

Eye Color Odds or Genetic Odds

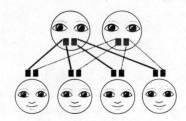

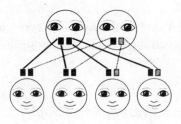

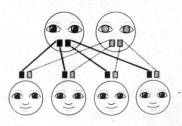

The odds are these combinations will not produce a blue-eyed baby.

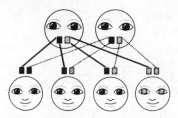

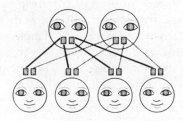

Two brown-eyed parents can produce a blue-eyed baby if they both are carriers of blue alleles. Although Mendel's Law predicts this couple is three times more likely to have a brown-eyed child, they may, in fact, have all blue-eyed babies.

Two blue-eyed parents are not likely to produce a brown-eyed baby.

This is a simplistic explanation of genetics. Of course, it doesn't always work as I've just described. To Mendel's laws, you must add these contingencies:

1. **Most traits are the result of several genes working together, called "polygenes."**
2. **All rules go out the window when genes mutate, or undergo a sudden, permanent, and often unexplained change. A classic example of such a mutation comes from Queen Victoria, a known carrier of the hemophilia gene. Because royalty lines are well documented, there is no evidence of any "bleeders" among her ancestors. It probably started as a gene mutation in the sperm or ovum of her parents.**

Remember that Mendel's laws deal only with probabilities. My father had brown eyes, my mother had blue. Because I ended up with blue eyes, we have to assume Dad carried one blue

allele. So the odds looked like this for my parents' four offspring:

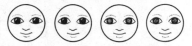

Instead, we ended up like this.

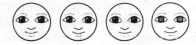

UNDER THE FAMILY TREE

Mendel studied how heredity plays a part in physical characteristics. Centuries later, we now know that genes are a factor in many serious diseases and even in personality.

Somewhere in our bodies are genes that predispose us to certain behavior, reactions, opinions, tastes, work habits, and more. We have all heard of those amazing studies of identical twins, separated at birth, who end up with similar likes and dislikes—even marrying similar spouses, sometimes with the same name!

When genetic traits combine with outside influences, it is easy to understand why each child turns out to be a wholly separate individual, with little genetic secrets that surface from time to time, causing parents to shake their heads and cry, "That's not *my* child!"

Though each of us gets half our genes from each parent, we are actually the sum total of many relatives and ancestors. Think about it: Half from each parent means 25 percent from each grandparent, and so on. The tree on page 17 shows how genes are shared.

GENE-SHARING ON YOUR FAMILY TREE

INSTRUCTION SHEET
FOUR GENERATION FAMILY TREE

① *Yourself*
② *Your Father*
③ *Your Mother*
④ *Your Father's Father (Grandfather)*
⑤ *Your Father's Mother (Grandmother)*
⑥ *Your Mother's Father (Grandfather)*
⑦ *Your Mother's Mother (Grandmother)*
⑧ *Your Father's Father's Father*
    (Great-grandfather)
⑨ *Your Father's Father's Mother*
    (Great-grandmother)
⑩ *Your Father's Mother's Father*
    (Great-grandfather)
⑪ *Your Father's Mother's Mother*
    (Great-grandmother)
⑫ *Your Mother's Father's Father*
    (Great-grandfather)

⑬ *Your Mother's Father's Mother*
    (Great-grandmother)
⑭ *Your Mother's Mother's Father*
    (Great-grandfather)
⑮ *Your Mother's Mother's Mother*
    (Great-grandmother)

Siblings, on the average, share 50% of same genes.

Only Identical Twins share 100% of same genes.

You get 50% of genes from each parent.
You get 25% of genes from each grandparent.

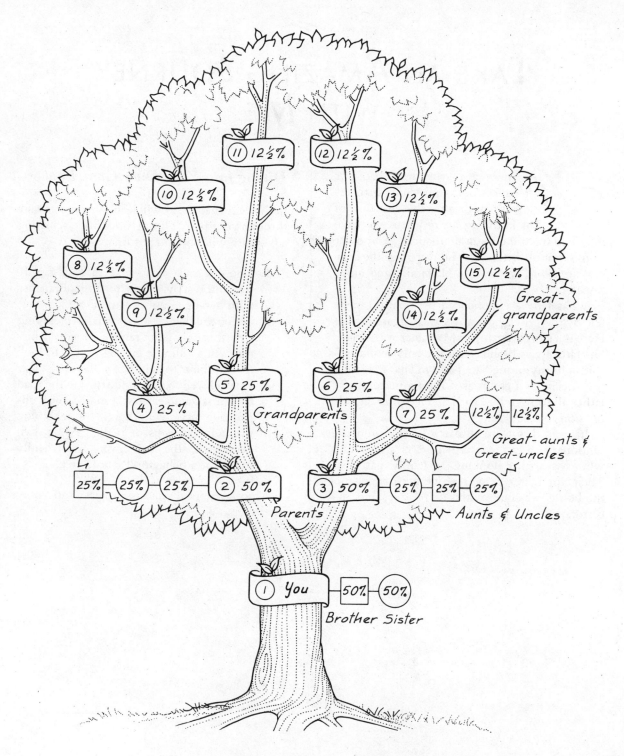

Gene-Sharing on Your Family Tree

TAKE AN AMAZING JOURNEY WITH ME

*K*nowing that we are part of our ancestors is not enough to re-affirm or alter the direction of our lives. But knowing *which* pieces we have inherited from them can dramatically empower us to savor our strengths and recognize the danger signals as we mature physically and emotionally.

What I have experienced personally can be felt by anyone who knows their genetic past. Here is a simple example: My father was blond. His father was blond. I am the only blond offspring in my immediate family. That made me feel special as a child, as if I got a piece of my father all to myself. That's an embarrassing admission, but it's the truth.

If, indeed, we are all part of a common evolutionary thread, we can more clearly define who we are by looking at family patterns. Then, for better or worse, we can understand the bonds we share with our relatives and ancestors.

Diving into Your Own Gene Pool

In the next chapters, I will lead you on a voyage through your past. This perilous but fascinating adventure will take three turns:

1. You'll learn how to make a basic family tree and discover how to fill its branches with eye-opening information.
2. Then, we'll take a potentially lifesaving trek through your family's medical history with a simple guide to what to look for and how to find it.
3. Finally, we'll come to the turn in the road that, if taken in earnest, can become a pilgrimage into your soul. I'll take you through the steps of making your own genogram, the first ever user-friendly model of a behavioral family tree.

Absorb yourself in this project, and enjoy the trip.

II

YOUR FAMILY TREE

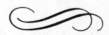

*There is a moral and philosophical
respect for our ancestors, which
elevates the character and improves
the heart.*
DANIEL WEBSTER

THE BEGINNINGS:
MAKING A BASIC FAMILY TREE

The United States is a rich and diverse land whose citizens have roots all over the world. However, tracing ancestry back to other lands can be complicated. For example, Jewish Americans might be unable to trace their line through the horrors of the Holocaust, when families were separated, records were obliterated, and relatives disappeared. And, as we learned in Alex Haley's *Roots*, the task is also difficult for African-Americans. They arrived in this land with virtually no family records intact, and families were usually broken apart by slavery. But every person should begin the search for ancestors in the same way—by gathering family stories, either from written records that are still available or by interviewing the oldest members of the clan.

Our Family Tree Workbook will focus on compiling the stories and backgrounds of ancestors who were already living on American soil. But I do offer some special resources for people of Jewish ancestry, African-Americans, Hispanics, Native Americans, and the families who arrived in this country from Asian lands. See Part V for special resources.

Any families who have been in this country for more than a generation do have some family tales that are quintessentially American. Next we will look at one example of how a devoted amateur genealogist unearthed her own family history.

The Story of Will Campbell

Sometime around 1875, William Clayton Campbell, the son of a blacksmith and wagon-maker from Polk County, Georgia, got into a scrape that changed his life forever.

It seems that Will was out for a stroll with his girlfriend when the town bully approached and hurled insults at the young lady. The two men argued, and before the obnoxious cad could spit out the wad of tobacco he was chewing, Will pulled out a gun and shot him dead.

But legend has it that the sheriff was a friend of the Campbell family and believed the town was better off with the bully dead. But he just couldn't let Will walk away free. So he told him to leave town and never come back. That is how Will Campbell ended up in Texas.

This became the secret scandal of the Campbell family from Georgia, and younger generations heard little about it. The women of the family, who in proper southern tradition kept track of such things, didn't talk about it and erased all signs of it from family records.

So one hundred years later, when Will's great-nephew Richard Campbell married Joyce Bates, the story of Will's overly eager trigger finger was all but lost when it came to conversations of family lore.

"Gran, Richard's mom, wouldn't tell us one thing," Joyce says. "But being from Georgia, we figured that anyone who fled to Texas was suspect."

The story might have stayed buried except that, years later, another family milestone came Joyce's way: Her first grandchild was born. She thought it would be a wonderful idea to surprise the family with a detailed baby book. Those of us who have lovingly labored over such books know they usually contain a simple family tree.

"That's when I realized I couldn't even remember the first name of one of my grand-mothers," says Joyce, who now lives on St. Simons Island off the coast of Georgia. "And I thought about all those people in my past and how I knew nothing about them." So Joyce set out on a journey of family discovery:

The first thing I did was talk to my oldest living relatives. I talked with Richard's relatives, too, so our children would have a full picture of their family tree from both sides. A friend of mine, who is an amateur genealogist, gave me some blank research sheets. Then I took a genealogy class at a local community college. Pretty soon, I was hooked.

After doing oral interviews with relatives, I went to local and country libraries. I learned where all the regional genealogical information was kept. With the librarian's help, I began to search for people with the same last names I saw on my family tree. I

figured if they came from the same county as my relatives, they were probably related, too. But I was looking for more than names and dates of birth. I wanted personalities, professions, happy and sad endings.

Some relatives wouldn't cooperate, or return phone calls. "That only made me more determined," says Joyce. "I learned about one dispute over funeral expenses years ago that left two sides of a family not speaking to each other. The youngest of the sisters from one side of the argument was still alive, but she refused to answer my questions. I guess I was descended from the wrong side." Joyce was in an odd situation, like a Hatfield courting a McCoy, seeking information instead of kisses:

So I went to the genealogical sections of libraries in places like Anniston, Alabama, and Owensboro, Kentucky, where I knew our ancestors had lived. I learned that other people—complete strangers—were researching the same family lines. They had left information and their addresses, and I began to write them letters.

I also left some information and my address at libraries. I joined the local genealogical societies and put queries in their bulletins. Sometimes I could get small local newspapers to do a short mention of my search.

I visited old cemeteries and searched their records. If I knew I was in a town where my ancestors had lived a generation or two back, I would find the oldest residents and interview them. You'd be amazed at the stories they could tell!

Soon my hard work really began to pay off. Mail came pouring in with stories about my ancestors. Some people even sent copies of obituaries from newspapers, and letters written by people decades ago. That's how I learned Richard came from a long line of rather opinionated newspaper publishers. In one town, someone angry at an editorial burned down the family's newspaper offices, but one ancestor found an alternative printing press and didn't miss an issue.

BECOMING A GENEALOGICAL SLEUTH: TIPS FROM JOYCE CAMPBELL

1. *Get information from the oldest family members right away. When they pass away, so do their secrets.*

2. *If a family member refuses to cooperate, it only makes the search more delicious. Usually it means a family scandal or something that used to be considered a delicate issue, like a disease or a criminal record.*

3. *Don't think of it as a search for just names and dates on a chart. Make them come alive with anecdotes and personality descriptions.*

Whatever Happened to Will?

Joyce Campbell eventually discovered that Will Campbell had been married in Texas, and every year he had written his mother, asking if it was safe for him to come back. "Every year, the answer was no," Joyce tells me. When his wife died forty years later, Will finally came back to Georgia.

"My oldest cousin was eight or nine when his elderly uncle Will came back from Texas," says Joyce. "He still remembers the stir that caused in the family." Will died in Georgia a short time later, but his family took him back to Greenville, Texas, for burial. His story would have died with him had Joyce Bates Campbell not jiggled the family tree and brought the facts back to life.

Joyce learned many other fascinating stories while researching her past—stories she will be able to pass on to future generations. Now, with Joyce as our inspiration, I will help you start your own search.

YOUR OWN FAMILY TREE WORKBOOK

This workbook will take you through the first two steps of our travels together: how to construct a family tree and where to find the necessary information. Think of the search as an archaeological dig, with the treasure being every gem of family history you can find.

Follow these step-by-step instructions and become an instant genealogist!

I. *THE MECHANICS OF A FAMILY TREE*

A. Decide on a family tree design (use a large sheet of paper).

There is no right or wrong way to design a family tree—it is as personal as bath soap. If you are a creative sort, you can come up with your own design. But there are three designs I consistently come across when looking through family history literature (see illustrations beginning page 25).

1. Artistic: This one actually looks like a tree, or is sometimes superimposed on a family coat of arms. It is the type of tree you are likely to find in a baby book or Bible. It is clever and decorative but offers little space for extra information. (See a sample artistic tree on page 25.)

2. Classic Block: These build from the bottom up, like an inverted pyramid. Squares represent males, circles represent females. Start with yourself as the "index person," indicated by a double square or double circle. Then connect yourself to a long horizontal line above your symbol. Add your siblings as squares or circles next to you and connect them to the line. Then extend a *T* shape from the center of the horizontal line, and add your parents (represented by a square and a circle) on either side of the *T*. This pattern can continue indefinitely. You can be creative with additional symbols, indicating marriage, divorce, remarriage, and other milestones. (Refer to the standardized symbols for a block graph found on page 26.)

(Note: This type of graph is usually used for medical family trees and genograms, which we'll discuss in later chapters.)

3. Standard Pedigree Chart: These charts read from left to right, and contain more information as you move to the right. These offer the most space for material but aren't as easy to read as the artistic tree. (See a sample pedigree chart on pages 30–31.)

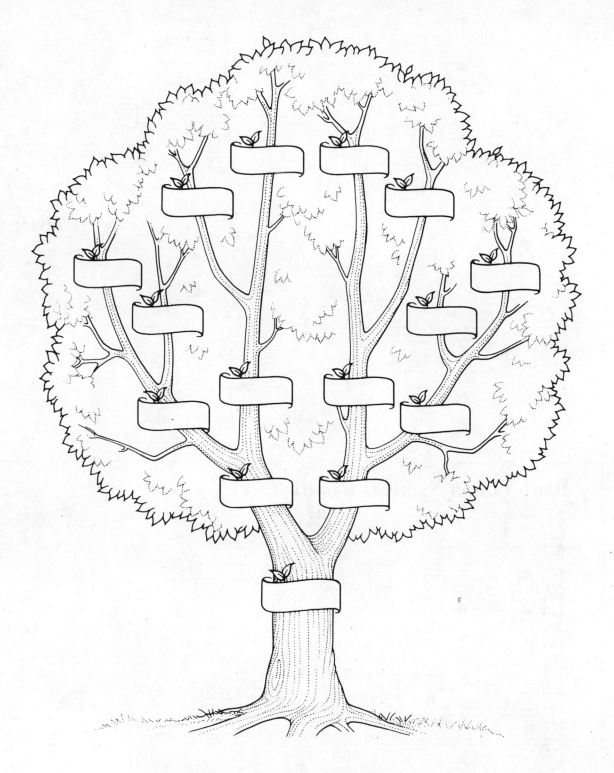

Artistic Family Tree

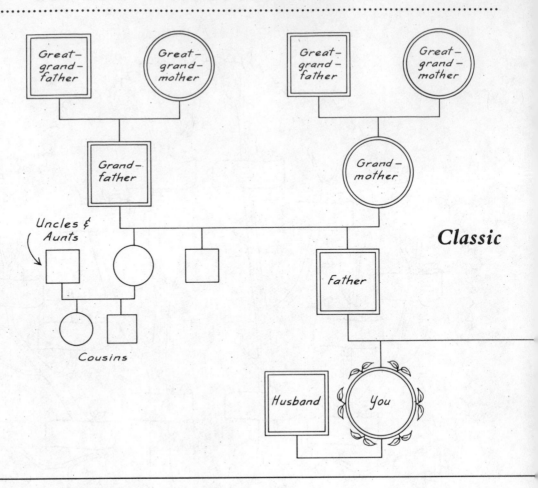

Classic

Block Graph Symbols Family Tree

standardized by the TASK FORCE OF THE NORTH AMERICAN PRIMARY CARE RESEARCH GROUP

☐ *Male*

◯ *Female*

▣ *"Index Person," Male* *

◉ *"Index Person," Female* *

☐——m. 1955——◯ *Marriage and Date (Year)*

☐——m. '48——d. '61——◯ *Married, Separated, Divorced and Dates*
(note : "19" omitted from dates – Include "18" for 1800's)

☐——m. '52——d. '60——◯——m. '64——◯ *Husband with more than one wife*

◯——m. '60——d. '67——☐——m. '69——d. '70——☐——m. '73——☐ *Wife with more than one husband*

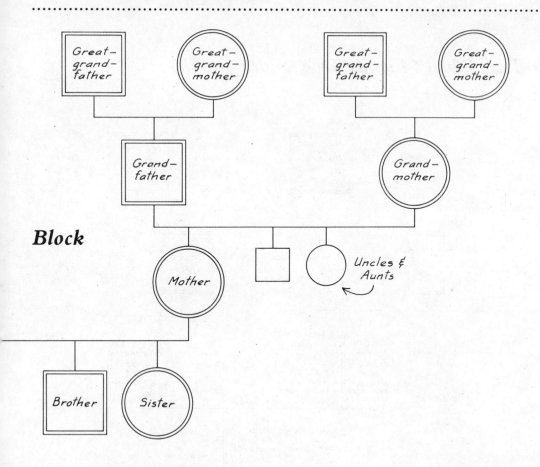

Block

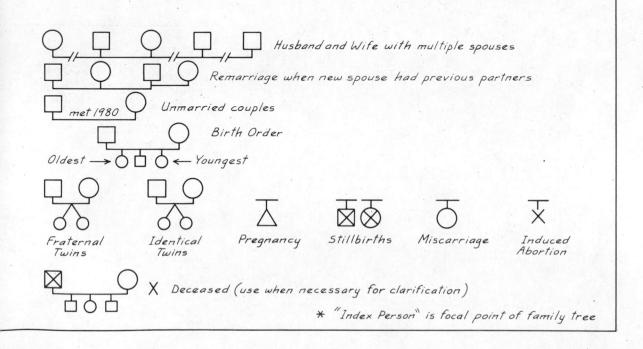

Husband and Wife with multiple spouses

Remarriage when new spouse had previous partners

met 1980   Unmarried couples

Birth Order

Oldest →   ← Youngest

Fraternal Twins   Identical Twins   Pregnancy   Stillbirths   Miscarriage   Induced Abortion

X   Deceased (use when necessary for clarification)

＊ "Index Person" is focal point of family tree

Richard Campbell's Family Tree (Block Graph)

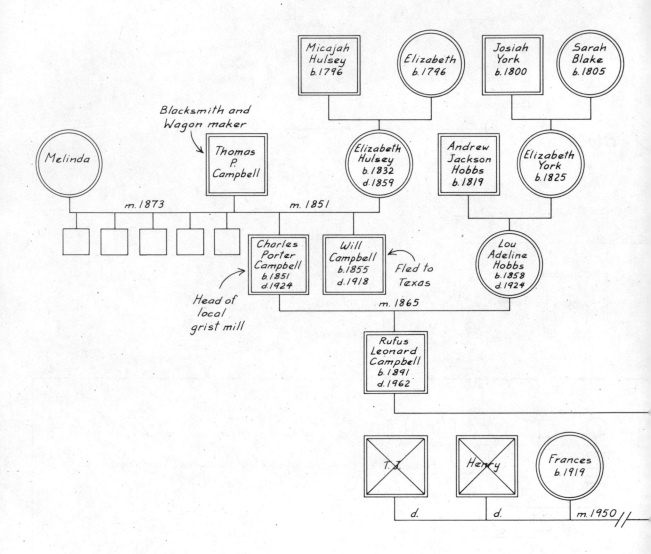

Courtesy of Joyce Bates Campbell

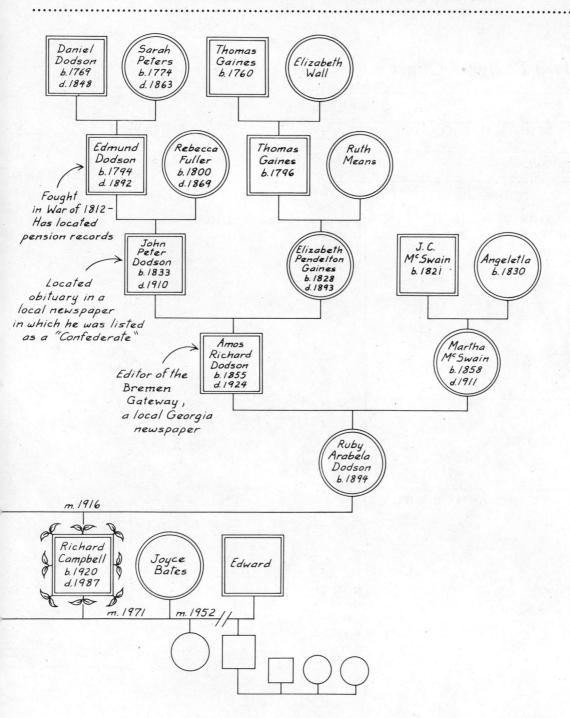

Daniel Dodson b.1769 d.1848

Sarah Peters b.1774 d.1863

Thomas Gaines b.1760

Elizabeth Wall

Edmund Dodson b.1794 d.1892

Rebecca Fuller b.1800 d.1869

Thomas Gaines b.1796

Ruth Means

Fought in War of 1812 – Has located pension records

John Peter Dodson b.1833 d.1910

Elizabeth Pendelton Gaines b.1828 d.1893

J.C. McSwain b.1821

Angeletla b.1830

Located obituary in a local newspaper in which he was listed as a "Confederate"

Editor of the Bremen Gateway, a local Georgia newspaper

Amos Richard Dodson b.1855 d.1924

Martha McSwain b.1858 d.1911

Ruby Arabela Dodson b.1894

m.1916

Richard Campbell b.1920 d.1987

Joyce Bates

Edward

m.1971   m.1952

Standard Pedigree Chart

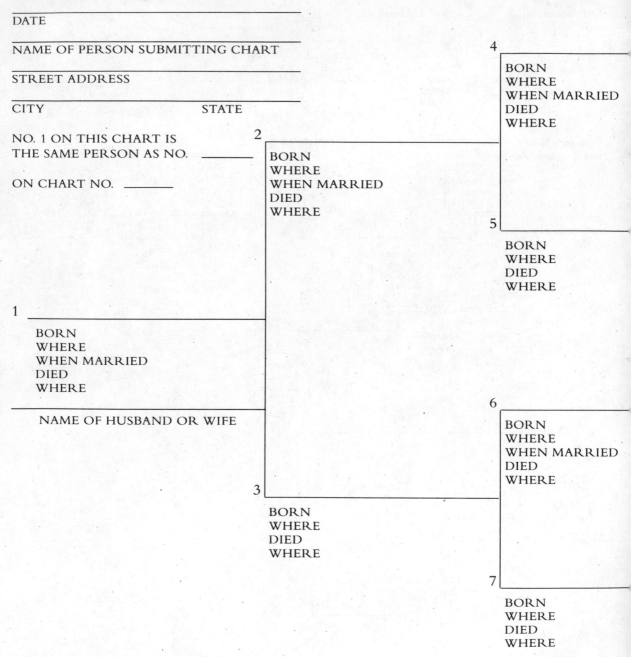

DATE

NAME OF PERSON SUBMITTING CHART

STREET ADDRESS

CITY   STATE

NO. 1 ON THIS CHART IS
THE SAME PERSON AS NO. _____

ON CHART NO. _____

2
BORN
WHERE
WHEN MARRIED
DIED
WHERE

4
BORN
WHERE
WHEN MARRIED
DIED
WHERE

5
BORN
WHERE
DIED
WHERE

1 _____
BORN
WHERE
WHEN MARRIED
DIED
WHERE

NAME OF HUSBAND OR WIFE

3
BORN
WHERE
DIED
WHERE

6
BORN
WHERE
WHEN MARRIED
DIED
WHERE

7
BORN
WHERE
DIED
WHERE

*Give here name of record or book where
this information was obtained. Refer to
names by number.*

CHART NO. ____

16

8

ABOVE NAME CONTINUES ON CHART
____

BORN
WHERE   17
WHEN MARRIED
DIED   ABOVE NAME CONTINUES ON CHART
WHERE   ____

18

9

ABOVE NAME CONTINUES ON CHART
____

BORN   19
WHERE
DIED   ABOVE NAME CONTINUES ON CHART
WHERE   ____

20

10

ABOVE NAME CONTINUES ON CHART
____

BORN   21
WHERE
WHEN MARRIED   ABOVE NAME CONTINUES ON CHART
DIED   ____
WHERE   22

11

ABOVE NAME CONTINUES ON CHART
____

BORN   23
WHERE
DIED   ABOVE NAME CONTINUES ON CHART
WHERE   ____

24

12

ABOVE NAME CONTINUES ON CHART
____

BORN   25
WHERE
WHEN MARRIED   ABOVE NAME CONTINUES ON CHART
DIED   ____
WHERE   26

13

ABOVE NAME CONTINUES ON CHART
____

BORN   27
WHERE
DIED   ABOVE NAME CONTINUES ON CHART
WHERE   ____

28

14

ABOVE NAME CONTINUES ON CHART
____

BORN   29
WHERE
WHEN MARRIED   ABOVE NAME CONTINUES ON CHART
DIED   ____
WHERE   30

15

ABOVE NAME CONTINUES ON CHART
____

BORN   31
WHERE
DIED   ABOVE NAME CONTINUES ON CHART
WHERE   ____

Pedigree Chart for Richard Campbell's Family

July 1990
DATE
Joyce Bates Campbell
NAME OF PERSON SUBMITTING CHART

STREET ADDRESS
St. Simons Island, Georgia
CITY   STATE

NO. 1 ON THIS CHART IS
THE SAME PERSON AS NO. ———

ON CHART NO. ———

1 *Richard Porter Campbell*

BORN   *1920*
WHERE *Polk Co., Georgia*
WHEN MARRIED *1950*
DIED   *1967*
WHERE *Cedartown, Georgia*
Joyce Bates
   NAME OF HUSBAND OR WIFE

2 *Rufus Leonard Campbell*

BORN   *May 14, 1891*
WHERE *Polk Co., Georgia*
WHEN MARRIED *Jan. 20, 1916*
DIED   *July 8, 1962*
WHERE *Rockmart, Ga.*

3 *Ruby Arabella Dodson*

BORN   *Feb. 12, 1894*
WHERE *Edwardsville, Alabama*
DIED
WHERE

4 *Charles Porter*

BORN   *Dec. 25,*
WHERE *Polk Co.,*
WHEN MARRIED
DIED   *Mar. 21,*
WHERE *Van Wert,*

5 *Lou Adeline*

BORN   *Oct. 10,*
WHERE *Polk Co.,*
DIED   *Nov. 9,*
WHERE *Van Wert,*

6 *Amos Richard*

BORN   *April 12,*
WHERE *Cleburne*
WHEN MARRIED
DIED   *Sept. 11,*
WHERE *Cleburne*

7 *Martha Josephine*

BORN   *Oct. 14,*
WHERE *Georgia*
DIED   *Aug. 20,*
WHERE *Buchanan*

Give here name of record or book where this information was obtained. Refer to names by number.

CHART NO. ____

16

8 Thomas P. Campbell

ABOVE NAME CONTINUES ON CHART

17

Campbell

BORN   around 1825
WHERE North Carolina
WHEN MARRIED 1851

ABOVE NAME CONTINUES ON CHART

1851
Ga.
Dec. 12, 1875

9

DIED   1904
WHERE Yorkville, Paulding Co.,
Elizabeth Hulsey   Ga.

18 Micajah (?) Hulsey

ABOVE NAME CONTINUES ON CHART

1923
Polk Co., Ga.

BORN   around 1832
WHERE
DIED   July 1, 1859
WHERE Polk Co., Ga.

19 Elizabeth

ABOVE NAME CONTINUES ON CHART

20

10 Andrew Jackson Hobbs

ABOVE NAME CONTINUES ON CHART

21

Hobbs

BORN   1819
WHERE
WHEN MARRIED
DIED
WHERE

ABOVE NAME CONTINUES ON CHART

1856
Ga.
1924
Polk Co.,
Ga.

11 Elizabeth York

22 Josiah York

ABOVE NAME CONTINUES ON CHART

BORN   1825
WHERE
DIED
WHERE

23 Sarah Virginia Blake

ABOVE NAME CONTINUES ON CHART

24 Edmond Dodson

ABOVE NAME CONTINUES ON CHART

12 John Peter Dodson

25 Rebecca Fuller

ABOVE NAME CONTINUES ON CHART

Dodson

BORN   Sept. 29, 1833
WHERE Alabama
WHEN MARRIED
DIED   June 1, 1911
WHERE Cleburne Co., Ala.

26 Thomas Gaines

ABOVE NAME CONTINUES ON CHART

1855
Co., Ala.
Nov. 7, 1875

13

Elizabeth Pendleton Gaines

27 Ruth Means

ABOVE NAME CONTINUES ON CHART

1924
Co., Ala.

BORN   June 23, 1828
WHERE Alabama
DIED   Oct. 13, 1893
WHERE Cleburne Co., Ala.

28

ABOVE NAME CONTINUES ON CHART

14 J. C. McSwain

29

McSwain

BORN   around 1829
WHERE Georgia
WHEN MARRIED
DIED
WHERE

ABOVE NAME CONTINUES ON CHART

1858

30

1911
–Harelson
Co., Ga.

15 Angeletta

ABOVE NAME CONTINUES ON CHART

BORN   1830
WHERE Kentucky
DIED
WHERE

31

ABOVE NAME CONTINUES ON CHART

B. Prepare blank sheets for extra information (see samples on following pages).
  1. Personal record sheets
  2. Family record sheets
C. Gather vital documents and papers
In particular, look for:
  1. Birth certificates. These contain date and location of birth and names of parents.
  2. Marriage licenses. These tell you when a whole new branch sprouted on your family tree.
  3. Divorce records
  4. Death certificates. These can supply critical death/medical information. They can also provide the name of the cemetery, which you can then contact for more records.
  5. Religious records
  a. Cemetery records. Do you think you know the name of the town where a relative died? Check the local cemeteries, find the date of death, and get a bonus: probably some interesting information about religion, family, and burial requests.
  b. Baptismal certificates, confirmation records, records of bar/bat mitzvahs.
  6. School information
  a. Report cards
  b. Yearbooks
  c. Graduation certificates
  d. Old textbooks
  7. Family papers
  a. Old driver's licenses
  b. Wills
  c. Insurance and banking records
  d. Diaries
  e. Address books
  f. Land grants and deeds, which can give you information about where ancestors lived and owned property. By looking up addresses, you can even visit old family homes.
  8. Military records, especially military pension files, which can tell you where an ancestor lived after years in the service,

---

DISCOVERING WHAT YOU DIDN'T KNOW ABOUT YOUR ETHNIC AND CULTURAL ROOTS

A friend of mine named Susan Silk, originally from Detroit, tells a captivating story about her Jewish ancestry. Her aunt recently gave her a box of old family documents, figuring Sue would be just the person to cull through them and see if they were of any importance.

Surprisingly, what Sue found were shares in a mine from Leadville, Colorado, dated 1892. The name on the shares: Mark Kahn, Sue's great-great-grandfather. Being a determined and curious person, Sue made a beeline to Leadville and found out the shares were still valid, but worthless, since that part of the mine was shut down. Or at least that's what she was told by the mining company, which was still very active in the area.

How did Mark get the shares? Sue learned that he saw opportunity in the burgeoning mining towns of Colorado and brought his wife and five children down from western Illinois to set up a general store. The miners would come into his shop for supplies, but had no cash. So they often would pay him in shares instead. It's a miniature slice of the multitextured Jewish-American story, and would have gone unnoticed by Sue's family if she had not begun a search into her ancestral history.

and whom he or she married. This could lead you to specific towns and cemeteries (you might even find some cousins you never knew you had!). You can also learn some fascinating "war stories."

9. Census records. These can tell you who lived in the same household as your ancestors.

10. Immigration records. Would you like to know where and when your family came to America? Immigration records can tell you this, plus how many people came over together, the names of their children, their country of origin, health status at arrival, their profession in the "old country," and much more.

II. *WHERE DO I FIND ALL THESE RECORDS AND DOCUMENTS?*

A. Vital Documents: birth, marriage, divorce, and death records

In Chapter V I list offices for vital documents in every state. These offices are listed as places to find death certificates (key information for your medical family tree), but staff there will also tell you where to find birth, marriage, and divorce records.

B. Religious Records

Is there a family Bible or other sacred text? Many records are handwritten right into the book. Contact officials at cemeteries, churches, temples, or any other place your ancestor may have worshiped and ask if they have records on anyone with your family name or names. You may have to try several sources before locating the one that was used by your ancestor. Much of this is guesswork. If you learn the name of the town where your ancestor was buried (from the death certificate or family stories), then contact houses of worship and cemeteries in that town.

C. School Information, Photos, and Other Family Papers

Contact schools and universities directly. Ask officials there how to get records on your ancestor. Each one has a policy for handling such requests.

Perhaps the most valuable source for school information is the family attic.

Check the dusty old trunks in the attics of your oldest relatives. You'd be amazed what you can find—yearbooks, pennants, football programs, and other clues to a life in decades past. (See sample letter for religious records and school information, page 42.)

D. Military Records

1. For ancestors in the service before World War I (1917)

   Write: The National Archives
   Reference Services Branch
   General Services Administration
   Washington, D.C. 20408

   (See sample letter, page 43.)

2. For ancestors who may have served after 1917

   Write: National Personnel Records
   Center
   Military Records Office
   NARA, 9700 Page Boulevard
   St. Louis, MO 63132

   (See sample letter, page 44.)

3. For ancestors who served during World War I (military draft registration records)

   Write: The National Archives
   Atlanta Branch
   1557 St. Joseph Avenue
   East Point, GA 30344

   (See sample letter, page 45.)

E. Census Documents

By law, these documents are kept confidential for seventy-two years after each census. Prior to 1900, records are rather sporadic, but if you know the names of ancestors who lived in this country from 1900 to 1920, you might be able to find some interesting information. (If you have ever filled out census forms, you know how much material they contain.)

Census copies are kept at The National Archives in Washington, D.C., and at twelve regional branches. For information on how to obtain census information, write to the Main Branch or branch nearest you.

(See sample letter, page 46.)
(For location of regional offices, see pages 165–66.)

MILITARY RECORDS REVEAL A SURPRISING SECRET

*M*ari, a friend and former neighbor of mine, is of Japanese descent. Her Japanese mother told her she had met her father, a white American, just after World War II and that he died shortly thereafter. She was raised by her mother and stepfather.

Her mother never spoke about Mari's biological father, and Mari somehow got the impression she wasn't supposed to ask about him. Recently, Mari was looking through some old photographs and saw a photo of her real father in a military uniform. She was able to determine the serial number on his shirt and had an inspiration: Why not find out where he was buried?

She called the public affairs office at a local military base, gave her father's serial number, and asked for burial information.

The person on the other end of the line came back with a surprising answer: "I have some good news and some bad news," he told her. "The good news is that your father is still alive. The bad news is that I'm not allowed to tell you where he is."

Once this startling news had sunk in, Mari asked if there was anything she was allowed

to know. "Well, I can tell you the location of the last veterans hospital he was treated at."

Without consulting her mother, Mari hired a private detective who very quickly came up with her father's address in Texas. She asked the detective to approach her father discreetly, so as not to disrupt the new family he had made since divorcing her mother.

The results were heartbreaking. He admitted his identity but denied he had ever been married to a Japanese woman or had had a daughter. Mari is still haunted by this sad rejection and now wonders if she should introduce herself to her three half-siblings, who probably don't even know she exists.

Mari wonders if she is a victim of postwar prejudice against the Japanese, which somehow scared off her father, making her mother so bitter she simply declared him dead. For now, Mari has decided not to confront her mother and wants to think over her next step. How sad that her true father might never know his daughter or granddaughter. But it is an example of how a little information can go a long way in searching for relatives and ancestors.

F. Immigration Records

There are several places where you might be able to find records of your immigrant ancestors:

1. *The National Archives.* If your ancestor arrived in the United States by ship after 1820, there might be a record of that arrival in The National Archives in Washington, D.C. If you know the name of your ancestor, the year and month of his or her arrival, and the name of the ship, the staff will search through their records for you. If you know only the name of your ancestor, you can go to the main branch of The National Archives or any regional branch and begin the search yourself. Ask for Form 81 to apply for a copy of the ship's manifest. (For addresses and phone numbers of National Archives Offices, see pages 165–66.)

(For sample letter, see page 47.)

2. *The U.S. Department of Justice.* For records from the Port of New York since 1897 (the arrival point for most immigrants) and other eastern seaboard ports since 1891 contact:

The United States Department of Justice
Immigration and Naturalization Service
Records and Verification Center
1446-21 Edwin Miller Boulevard
Martinsburg, W.V 25401

(For sample letter, see page 48.)

3. *The Genealogical Society of Utah.* This unparalleled resource has a computerized index of 60 million immigrants in its Family History Library. There are over a thousand branches of the library.

To find the location nearest you, call the local Mormon Church (listed in the phone book under the "Church of Jesus Christ of Latter-Day Saints") or write the central library:

Family History Library
35 North West Temple Street
Salt Lake City, UT 84150

4. *The Immigration and Naturalization Service.* If your ancestor became a citizen after 1906, there's probably a record of him or her at the INS Office. Contact the Immigration and Naturalization Service and make a request under the Freedom of Information Act/Privacy Act. Ask for Form G-639. (The form is an application for immigration records.) Write:

Immigration and Naturalization Service
FOIA/PA Office
Washington, D.C. 20536

(For sample letter, see page 49.)

G. Oral Histories

Get out a tape recorder and talk to your relatives, especially the oldest ones. They should be full of wonderful anecdotes and tips on where to look next. Family photographs are a particularly useful tool to prompt the memory, often leading to the recollection of long-forgotten—and often valuable—details. Be especially curious if a relative refuses to discuss someone or something in the past. (More on this in the workbook section of Part III.)

H. Written Family Histories

Write as many relatives as possible informing them of whatever preliminary work you've done, and ask them to add or correct your family-tree-in-progress. They could be your most valuable resource.

Sample: Personal Record (for   )

Sources:

NAME:

BIRTHPLACE (City, County, State)

FATHER'S NAME:

MOTHER'S MAIDEN NAME:

MARRIAGE:
To:

Date: Place:

CHILDREN:
Name: Born: Date   Born: Place

DATE OF BIRTH:

HOMES:

OCCUPATION:

EDUCATION:

RELIGION:

DEATH:
Date: Place:

Burial Place:

Sample: Personal Record (for My Grandfather)

NAME: ERNST JOHN HENRY KRAUSE   DATE OF BIRTH: July 21, 1882

BIRTHPLACE (City, County, State)   Germany

FATHER'S NAME: Ernst Krause Sr.

MOTHER'S MAIDEN NAME: Bertha Braun

MARRIAGE:
To: Martha Louise Auguste Strege
Date: Nov. 6, 1907   Place: Milwaukee, Wis.

CHILDREN:

Name	Date Born:	Place Born:
Arthur Ernst	Aug. 13, 1908	Milwaukee
Bertha H.	May 23, 1910	'' (d. 1942)
Ernst Henry Phillip	May 2, 1913	''
Walter A.	Aug. 1, 1914	'' (d. 1969)
Henry John	Jan. 17, 1916	''

HOMES: Came to U.S. at age 9 months on SS Braunschweig from Bremen, arriving in Baltimore on June 14, 1883.[1] Settled in Milwaukee. Naturalized Sept. 26, 1906.[2]

OCCUPATION: Chef–Pfister Hotel, Athletic Club (Milwaukee)

EDUCATION:

RELIGION: Trinity Ev. Luth. Church, Milwaukee

DEATH:
Date: March 26, 1916   Place: Milwaukee, Wis.

Burial
Place: Union Cemetery. Later Moved to Graceland Cemetery.

Was a baker by the age of 17.[3]

Baked the wedding cake for wedding of half-sister Martha to Otto Zellmer.[4]

May have gone to other cities such as St. Louis to work.

Probably met his wife at the Strege home, where he had been invited because his sisters did domestic work with Katie Masch, who later married Frank Strege.[5]

Met Martha Strege earlier than September 7, 1907.[6]

Son Arthur Krause has a table that was his.

Son Ernst Krause has a French gourmet cookbook that was his.

Son Henry has a gold pocket watch that was his.

Sources:
Source is Arthur E. Krause if not otherwise stated.
1 Ship's List, SS Braunschweig, arrived in Baltimore on June 14, 1883
2 Certificate of Naturalization
3 Census, 1900, Milwaukee, Vol. 52, E.D. 181, Sheet 1
4 Martha Zellmer, 1979
5 Katie Strege, 1980
6 Love letter of EJHK to Martha Strege, Sept. 7, 1907

NAME _____ **FAMILY RECORD SHEET** Child No. in Family . . . . .

Give Name In Full If Female Give Maiden Name

	Day	Month	Year	City	County	State	FATHER
Born							Born
Married							Died
Died							MOTHER
Buried							Born
Church			Occupation				Died

MARRIED To.

Give Name In Full If Female Give Maiden Name

	Day	Month	Year	City	County	State	FATHER
Born							Born
Died							Died
Buried							MOTHER
Church							Born
If Married Twice Name of Second Spouse							Died

Born	Married	Died	No. Children

SEX	Give Full Name of Child In order of birth		Day	Month	Year	City	County	State
1		Born						
		Died						
	Married To	Married						
		Born						
		Died						
2		Born						
		Died						
	Married To	Married						
		Born						
		Died						
3		Born						
		Died						
	Married To	Married						
		Born						
		Died						
4		Born						
		Died						
	Married To	Married						
		Born						
		Died						
5		Born						
		Died						
	Married To	Married						
		Born						
		Died						
6		Born						
		Died						
	Married To	Married						
		Born						
		Died						
7		Born						
		Died						
	Married To	Married						
		Born						
		Died						

Give as much information as possible about each person, characteristics, life work.

| NAME | Thomas P. CAMPBELL | | | | **FAMILY RECORD SHEET** | | Child No. in Family . . . . . |

Give Name In Full If Female Give Maiden Name

	Day	Month	Year	City	County	State	FATHER
Born		circa 1825-1831				N.C.	Born
Married							Died
Died							MOTHER
Buried				Yorkville Cemetery-Paulding G.			Born
Church	Beulah Baptist		Occupation Blacksmith, wagon maker, farmer				Died

MARRIED To. Elizabeth (Lizbeth) HULSEY

Give Name In Full If Female Give Maiden Name

	Day	Month	Year	City	County	State	FATHER
Born		1834			Paulding	GA.	Born Micajah HULSEY 1794
Died				Van Wert	Polk	GA.	Died
Buried	age: 27			Van Wert	PLK	GA.	MOTHER Elizabeth 1796
Church	Van Wert Methodist Cemetery						Born
If Married Twice Name of Second Spouse Malinda HEATON							Died

| Born | Paulding Co. | Married | | Died | Yorkville Cemetery 14 Dec. 1907 | No. Children 5 |

SEX	Give Full Name of Child In order of birth			Day	Month	Year	City	County	State
1	Charles Porter CAMPBELL	Born		25	Dec.	1851			
		Died		21	Mar.	1923	Van Wert	Polk	GA.
	Married To Lou Adeline HOBBS	Married		12	Dec.	1875	W.W. Simpson	Polk	GA.
		Born		10	Oct.	1856			
		Died		9	Nov.	1924			
2	(Clayton) William C. CAMPBELL	Born							
		Died							
	Married To	Married							
		Born							
		Died				1918	Greenville		Texas
3	John F. CAMPBELL	Born		13	Dec.	1867			
		Died		27	Jan.	1944	Beulah	Pauld.	GA.
	Married To Sallie VERNER	Married							
		Born							
		Died							
4	James Oscar CAMPBELL	Born		2	Aug.	1874			
		Died		3	Dec.	1943	Beulah	Pauld.	GA.
	Married To Lucy Ann	Married							
		Born		6	Jul.	1874			
		Died		5	Jun.	1962			
5	Frank CAMPBELL	Born							
		Died					Yorkville	Pauld.	GA.
	Married To Rudy	Married							
		Born							
		Died					Yorkville	Pauld.	GA.
6	Felton CAMPBELL	Born							
		Died							
	Married To	Married							
		Born							
		Died							
7	Wiley S. CAMPBELL	Born		7	Oct.	1879			
		Died		25	Dec.	1950	Beulah	Pauld.	GA.
	Married To Dovie GAMEL	Married							
		Born							
		Died							

mother of 5 sons

Give as much information as possible about each person, characteristics, life work.

Sample Letter:

To Be Sent to: Places of Worship, Cemeteries, Schools, and Universities

---

```
                                    Grace Doe
                                    23 Main Street
                                    Seaport, MN 55440
                                    612-555-2950


                                    9/9/93


The Everlasting Peace Cemetery
1234 Dove Drive
Faith, SD 54321

To the Director:


    I represent the Doe family of Seaport, Minnesota. We are
currently doing genealogical research and are looking for
information on an ancestor who might (be buried in your
cemetery/have been a member of your church/have attended your
school).
    We believe that my great-aunt Sylvia Doe Burke died in your
town around 1957 and (attended your church/school, etc.). We
would very much appreciate the following information:
    1. Do your records show a person with that name?
    2. How can I obtain copies of her (church, burial, or
       school) records?
    Please be assured that this information is for genealogical
purposes only. I very much appreciate any help you can give us.
I have enclosed a self-addressed, stamped envelope.


                                    Waiting to hear from you,



                                    (Your signature)

                                    Grace Doe
```

Sample Letter:

Sending for Military Records Before 1917

```
                                    Your Name
                                    Your Address
                                    Your Daytime Phone

                                    Date


The National Archives
Reference Services Branch
General Services Administration
Washington, D.C. 20408


To Whom It May Concern:

    I represent the (family name) of (city, state). We are
currently doing genealogical research and hope you can help us.
We are looking for information about _____, our
ancestor who served in the military in (the era or approximate
year).
    We would like copies of all military and pension records on
_____. We believe he was born around (year),
possibly in (city, state).
    Please let me know how I can obtain these copies. Please
also send me the NATF Form 80 for Copies of Veterans Records, so
I can request the assistance of your staff in this research. I
am enclosing a self-addressed, stamped envelope.


                                    Thank you,



                                    Your signature

                                    Your printed name
```

Sample Letter:

Sending for Military Records After 1917

Your Name
Your Address
Your Daytime Phone

Date

National Personnel Records Center
Military Records Office
NARA, 9700 Page Boulevard
St. Louis, MO 63132

To Whom It May Concern:

I represent the (family name) family of (city, state). We are currently doing genealogical research on our family and are interested in locating records about an ancestor who served in the military during (indicate which war).

His name is _____. He was born in (year) in (city, state). We would like copies of all military and pension records of _____. Please let me know how to obtain these copies.

I have enclosed a self-addressed, stamped envelope for your convenience.

Thank you very much.

Your signature

Your printed name

Sample Letter:

For 1917 Military Draft Registration Records

                                        Your Name
                                        Your Address
                                        Your Daytime Phone

                                        Date

The National Archives
Atlanta Branch
1557 St. Joseph Avenue
East Point, GA 30344

To Whom It May Concern:

   I represent the (family name) family of (city, state). We
are currently doing genealogical research and are interested in
locating all military and pension records of (ancestor's name),
who served in World War I. He was born in (year) in (city,
state).
   Please let me know how to obtain copies of draft
registration and other military records of _____.
                                                  (name)
   I have enclosed a self-addressed, stamped envelope for your
convenience.

                                        Thank you very much,

                                        Your signature

                                        Your printed name

Sample Letter:

To Send for Census Records. (Note: No self-addressed envelope is needed.)

                                        Your Name
                                        Your Address
                                        Your Daytime Phone

                                        Date

The National Archives
(Choose address of branch nearest you.
 For address, see pages 165-66.)

Dear Census Officials:

    I represent the (family name) family of (city, state). We
are currently doing genealogical research and would like to
locate census records for our ancestor, _____, who
                                              (name)
was the head of his household in (city, state) in (year). He
arrived _____.
               (date)
    Please send me information on how to find and use census
records.

                                        Thank you,

                                        Your signature

                                        Your printed name

Sample Letter:

To Send for Immigration Records (if relative arrived in the U.S. by ship after 1820).

```
                                    Your Name
                                    Your Address
                                    Your Daytime Phone

                                    Date


The National Archives
General Reference Branch
Eighth Street and Pennsylvania Avenue, NW
Washington, D.C. 20408


To Whom It May Concern:

     I represent the (family name) family of (city, state). We
are currently doing genealogical research and are trying to
locate immigration records on our ancestor. He (first name) and
his wife (first name) arrived by ship at the Port of New York in
the spring of (year). Please inform me of how I can learn the
name of their ship.
     Please send me Form 81 to apply for a copy of the ship's
manifest. Please let me know of any fees for this service.


                              Thank you,



                              Your signature

                              Your printed name
```

Sample Letter:

To Send for Immigration Records (if relative arrived at Port of New York since 1897 or other eastern seaboard ports since 1891).

```
                              Your Name
                              Your Address
                              Your Daytime Phone

                              Date

The United States Department of Justice
Immigration and Naturalization Service
 Records and Verification Center
1446-21 Edwin Miller Boulevard
Martinsburg, WV 25401

To Whom It May Concern:

    I represent the (family name) family of (city, state). We
are currently doing genealogical research and are seeking
immigration records for our ancestor, _____, who
                                            (name)
came to the Port of New York from (country) in (year). Please
send me FORM G-641 so I may apply for her records. I would
appreciate any additional information on how I may obtain
immigration records for our ancestor.

                              Thank you,


                              Your signature

                              Your printed name
```

Sample Letter:

To Send for Immigration and Naturalization (Citizenship) Records after 1906

```
                              Your Name
                              Your Address
                              Your Daytime Phone

                              Date


Immigration and Naturalization Service
FOIA/PA Office
Washington, D.C. 20536


To Whom It May Concern:

     I represent the (family name) family of (city, state). We
would like to find copies of the naturalization papers of our
ancestor, _____.
     Please send us Form G-639 as we would like to apply for
these records under the Freedom of Information Act/Privacy Act.
     Thank you,



                              Your signature

                              Your printed or typed name
```

STEPPING FOOT ON AMERICAN SOIL

*I*f your family arrived in America at the height of the immigration years (1820–1920), he or she arrived by boat. You might find records in the port city.

The vast majority of immigrants came through Ellis Island. It was nicknamed the "Isle of Hope and Tears" because it wasn't until immigrants arrived that they learned if they could stay or would be sent back (usually because of poor health).

A visit to the island, near the Statue of Liberty in New York Harbor, can be a moving experience. There is a library and museum there housing special collections of photographs, clippings, books, and periodicals—but no immigration records.

The National Park Service has plans to open what it will call the Ellis Island Family History Center sometime in the next few years. It is an ambitious project, with plans to computerize details about the more than 17 million immigrants who passed through the Isle of Hope and Tears from 1892 all the way to 1957. It will also include records dating from 1850–92, when immigrants were processed at Castle Clinton, a building in New York's Battery district.

The proposed Family History Center will have thirty-two computers for people to research their ancestors. The Ellis Island Restoration Committee is now in the final fundraising process for this exciting venture.

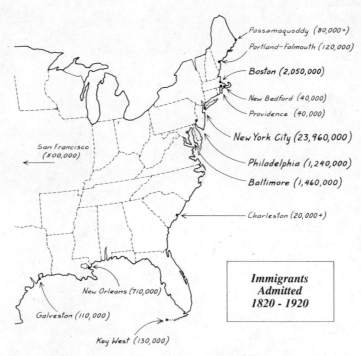

Passamaquoddy (80,000+)
Portland–Falmouth (120,000)
Boston (2,050,000)
New Bedford (40,000)
Providence (40,000)
New York City (23,960,000)
Philadelphia (1,240,000)
Baltimore (1,460,000)
Charleston (20,000+)
San Francisco (500,000)
New Orleans (710,000)
Galveston (110,000)
Key West (130,000)

Immigrants Admitted 1820 - 1920

Based on Information from Statue of Liberty / Ellis Island National Monument, National Park Service.

WHAT'S NEXT?

genealogical search is endless and often addictive. But once you have some basic information on your family tree, you are ready for the next step; the search for medical information.

This detective work is more than fascinating—it could be lifesaving. The next part will provide step-by-step information on how you can learn more about the potential—good and bad—beneath your skin. And we will learn how this information can empower you to take control of your physical well-being.

THE FASCINATING FUTURE OF DNA FINGERPRINTING

he legal maneuverings in the O. J. Simpson murder trial have made us aware of the power of genetic evidence in criminal cases. Since its first use in the United States in 1987, DNA fingerprinting has been employed in nearly 25,000 cases. Newsweek magazine reports that in one-third of these cases, DNA evidence has actually cleared people mistakenly suspected of crimes. DNA evidence has proved the innocence of at least a dozen men in prison for brutal crimes, and they were eventually freed. And in April 1994, Virginia had the first execution of a murderer convicted on DNA evidence.

To produce a DNA fingerprint, lab technicians take a DNA sample from hair, blood, or semen and put it through a process that results in a series of parallel lines of varied thickness, with bulges, dots, and dashes along the line. This is a far more detailed and precise image than those produced by traditional tests, and is considered to be far more reliable. Most experts say that the odds against a false DNA match approach one in a million, although there are a few scientists (and defense lawyers) who dispute that estimate.

There is no question that in the future many criminal cases will be decided by the physical evidence produced by the fascinating, microscopic material within our bodies. While the accuracy of tests can be debated, DNA is unique to every individual (with the exception of identical twins) and can reveal the truth.

III

YOUR MEDICAL
FAMILY TREE

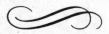

Accidents occur in the best regulated families.
CHARLES DICKENS,
DAVID COPPERFIELD

GROWING A TREE OF LIFE AND HEALTH: MAKING YOUR MEDICAL FAMILY TREE

We are shocked when a forty-year-old friend gets cancer or dies of a heart attack. But the clues to these tragedies could have been in clear sight on their medical family trees, screaming to be noticed. As a culture, we are only beginning to understand how family plays a part in our future health, and we are even less informed about reading and heeding the warning signs that could help save our lives.

This chapter will give you the tools you need to learn how the odds stack up for you in your quest for a long life. You will learn how to build your medical family tree, branch by branch, until you have a clear picture of how genetics might impact you. This is important for two reasons: (1) If you know you are at high risk for a certain illness, your doctor can be more aggressive with your regular check-ups and be better equipped to catch problems early enough for successful treatment. (2) If you are about to start a family of your own, a medical family tree will help you make some family-planning decisions. Your doctor will thank you for gathering your family medical history! But most of all, you will thank yourself.

Inherited Childhood Diseases

Over 15 million Americans suffer from inherited diseases. The Hereditary Disease Foundation in Santa Monica, California, says genetic illnesses account for one-third of all childhood hospitalizations, almost half of all infant deaths, and an even larger number of miscarriages, and many cases of mental retardation.

For this reason, the study of genetics and disease in medical school has traditionally been left to pediatricians-in-training. For years, most inherited diseases were believed to surface in childhood. Among the most common ones are:

Cystic fibrosis
Tay-Sachs disease
Hemophilia
Duchenne muscular dystrophy
Sickle-cell anemia
Thalassemia (form of anemia)
Common form of Down's syndrome
Certain birth defects
Some types of dwarfism and short stature
Retinoblastoma (eye tumor)

When children are diagnosed with a hereditary disease or problem, the family usually gets swallowed up in the unrelenting medical system that cares for the life of the child. The good news in all of this is that those families have an opportunity to receive helpful genetic counseling.

But many adult diseases, especially heart disease and cancer, are beginning to surprise us with the extent of their genetic links. It was only in 1980, for example, that Dr. M. Steven Piver of the newly renamed Gilda Radner Familial Ovarian Cancer Registry in Buffalo, New York, began to discover the insidious family connection with some ovarian cancers.

In fact, it is believed that there are almost five thousand hereditary illnesses, some of them extremely rare. This chapter will focus on the most common inherited diseases in adulthood, but what you will learn about making your family medical tree can be applied to any disease. You will simply be looking for a suspicious pattern.

Because the role of genetics in adult illness is still not emphasized in medical schools in this country, it is safe to say that most family doctors do not fully understand the clues. Some physicians might be offended by this statement, but as you learned from my family's story, I, unfortunately, have considerable personal experience with this problem.

Why Do I Want to Know About My Possible Medical Fate?

This is a provocative question indeed. As scientists get more clever at unraveling family medical links, some families are asking: "Why would we want to know?" This is an especially difficult question for families with histories of untreatable diseases. We learned more about the devastation of Huntington's chorea when folk singer Woody Guthrie was stricken. Many wondered if his son, singer Arlo Guthrie, would also be hit. (Arlo has a 50 percent chance of getting this illness, in which the body and mind slowly deteriorate.)

Some family members at high risk for diseases like Huntington's chorea choose not to be tested, believing that not knowing is better than finding out for certain that they will get it. Others are locked in uncertainty, because no test is available for their family's particular strain of disease.

But for diseases that can be short-circuited with intervention, we face altogether different issues. For some of us, it is tempting to look the other way, to avoid what we see as more sources of anxiety in our already overstressed lives. A century, a half century, even two decades ago, this would have been an understandable option.

But medical technology is exploding in a way that empowers us to change our fate. Can you look the other way when it may be within your power to save, or prolong, your own life? You may have heard of this new scientific research under a simple umbrella term: gene therapy.

Do You Have to Live with the Genes You Were Born With?

Just recently, the United States became the first nation to allow new genes to be introduced into people. The first gene therapy on an already born human being began in September 1990 at the National Institutes of Health. A four-year-old girl was suffering from adenosine enzyme deficiency (ADA), which wipes out the immune system (like the Houston boy who died after leaving his protective "bubble").

NIH doctors took her own white blood cells, multiplied them in the laboratory, added the missing ADA gene, and put the altered fluid back into her body. Three years later, she was doing fine.

Gene Therapy for Cancer

Experiments have also been tried with a handful of cancer patients who, it is hoped, will benefit from genetically altered tumor-fighting white blood cells. It was first tried with success on two people with advanced melanoma (skin cancer). Then, in early 1993, NIH approved a gene-therapy experiment for a severely ill woman with a brain tumor. Doctors gave the fifty-one-year-old patient injections of her own cells after they took them out and genetically altered them. This was done in the hope they would stimulate her own immune system to fight the cancer cells. Months later, the woman was holding her own, long after she was expected to die. Gene therapy gave her an unprecedented and unexpected gift of a longer life.

But, remember, this was a last-ditch effort to help a dying patient after all other conventional treatments failed. The full impact of this kind of medical treatment will not be known until healthier patients are injected with genetically altered cells.

Gene Therapy and Heart Disease

This unique approach to treatment could also lead to dramatic help for people who inherited heart problems. Suppose you were born without the precious gene that helps to take the bad cholesterol out of the blood. This leads to a genetic condition called hypercholesterolemia, or severely high levels of the "bad" cholesterol.

If gene therapy advances the way doctors hope, the missing gene could be put into the patient's body. If it works, cholesterol could miraculously be restored to normal levels, protecting the patient from an almost certain early death from heart disease.

Other Possibilities for Gene Therapy

So far, scientists have learned only how to introduce a single gene into an ill body. But many

WHAT DOES EACH GENE DO? THE HUMAN GENOME PROJECT MIGHT SOON TELL US!

*E*very now and then we read an article about a highly touted discovery of a gene linked to some disease. We're never quite sure what it means, and it only makes the connection between our bodies and genetics more confusing.

For example, scientists think they have found the culprit gene in a certain form of hereditary colon cancer. But it has little impact on another form of inherited colon cancer. Scientists think they have found a gene linked to alcoholism. But what about the obvious environmental factors that contribute to the disease?

And why have they found genes linked to certain ailments but not to others? A decade from now we might not be asking these questions.

Scientists from all over the world are now involved in a massive undertaking to chart, or map, each gene and its function. (So far, they have identified only about three thousand of the one hundred thousand human genes.) It is called the Human Genome Project, a gene treasure hunt of sorts that will cost 3 billion dollars. The target date for completion is the year 2004. Recently, scientists on the gene-mapping project announced they have made the first comprehensive charts for two of the body's twenty-three chromosomes: the "Y" chromosome, which specifies the maleness of an embryo, and the notorious "Chromosome 21," linked to disorders like Down's syndrome and Alzheimer's disease.

Some of the biggest names in biology are involved in this project, and they hope eventually to decode the information on each gene—more specifically, the genetic instructions encoded on 3 billion pairs of proteins that make up human DNA. Sound complicated?

We'll let the scientists worry about the details. What we should know about this project is that it could have a revolutionary impact on the way we diagnose, treat, and even prevent disease. Identifying the function of each gene won't cure every inherited disease, but it will give scientists clear targets for treatment. Some ethicists worry that research will lead to abuses and unneeded tinkering with our genetic blueprints, but it is giving hope to millions whose children are at risk for inherited problems.

Krause Medical Family Tree (Spouses Not Included)

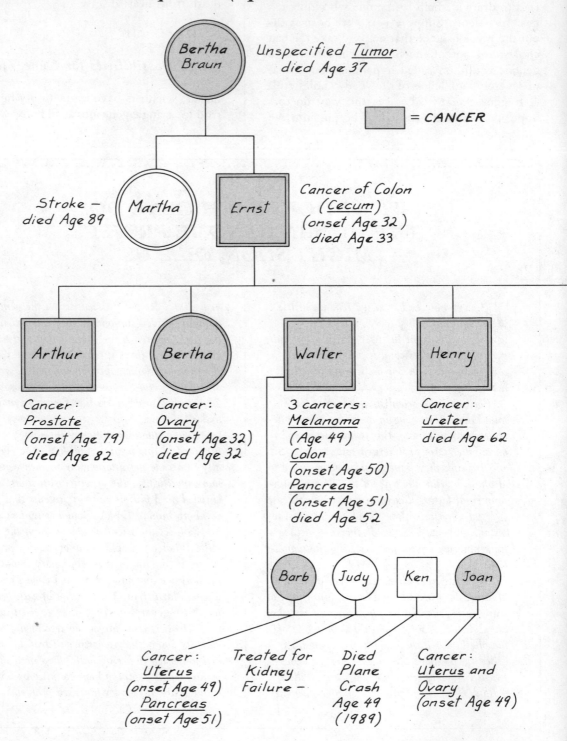

Bertha Braun — Unspecified *Tumor* died Age 37

☐ = *CANCER*

Stroke — died Age 89 — Martha

Ernst — Cancer of Colon (*Cecum*) (onset Age 32) died Age 33

Arthur — Cancer: *Prostate* (onset Age 79) died Age 82

Bertha — Cancer: *Ovary* (onset Age 32) died Age 32

Walter — 3 cancers: *Melanoma* (Age 49) *Colon* (onset Age 50) *Pancreas* (onset Age 51) died Age 52

Henry — Cancer: *Ureter* died Age 62

Barb — Cancer: *Uterus* (onset Age 49) *Pancreas* (onset Age 51)

Judy — Treated for Kidney Failure —

Ken — Died Plane Crash Age 49 (1989)

Joan — Cancer: *Uterus* and *Ovary* (onset Age 49)

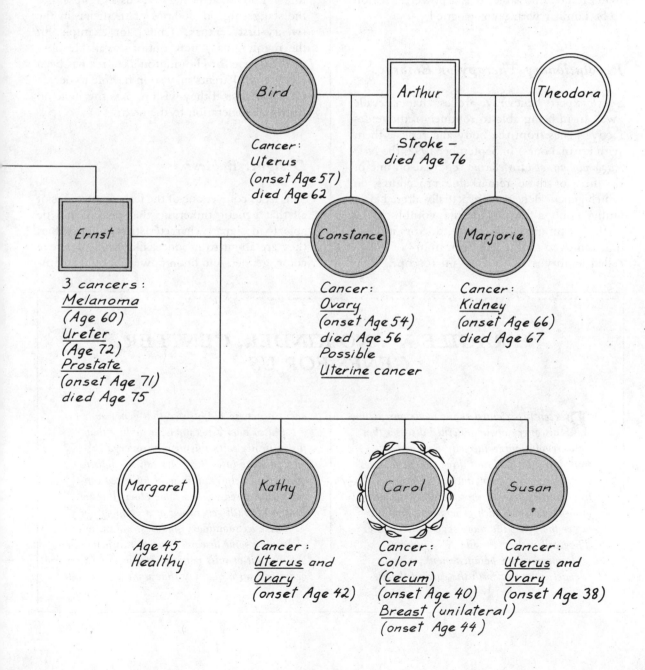

Bird

Cancer:
<u>Uterus</u>
(onset Age 57)
died Age 62

Arthur

Stroke –
died Age 76

Theodora

Ernst

3 cancers:
<u>Melanoma</u>
(Age 60)
<u>Ureter</u>
(Age 72)
<u>Prostate</u>
(onset Age 71)
died Age 75

Constance

Cancer:
<u>Ovary</u>
(onset Age 54)
died Age 56
Possible
<u>Uterine</u> cancer

Marjorie

Cancer:
<u>Kidney</u>
(onset Age 66)
died Age 67

Margaret

Age 45
Healthy

Kathy

Cancer:
<u>Uterus</u> and
<u>Ovary</u>
(onset Age 42)

Carol

Cancer:
Colon
(<u>Cecum</u>)
(onset Age 40)
<u>Breast</u> (unilateral)
(onset Age 44)

Susan

Cancer:
<u>Uterus</u> and
<u>Ovary</u>
(onset Age 38)

diseases are caused by a mischievous mixture of genes, either too many of the wrong genes or not enough of the right ones. Geneticists are looking to future years, when they will be able to determine what combination of genes can be introduced or eliminated from humans to attack more complicated diseases.

Gene therapy could revolutionize the way we treat many illnesses, because it uses the patient's own body as medicine, the most custom-made remedy possible. It is a powerful reason to be familiar with your genetic legacy.

Revolutionary Therapy on Embryos

Some experts believe we are less than a decade away from being able to routinely remove defective genes from the body and replace them with normal ones. In September 1992, the *New England Journal of Medicine* reported on one of the first of these remarkable procedures, in which genetic defects were actually altered in an embryo only a few days in the womb!

In that futuristic procedure, doctors in London removed single cells from four- or eight-celled embryos. Under a microscope, they looked for genes known to cause cystic fibrosis. Embryos found to have the always-fatal disorder were discarded, and the others were reinserted into the mother's expanding uterus.

Removing a single cell did not appear to harm the healthy embryos. The first child tested this way was born without incident and, as tested, does not have cystic fibrosis.

Putting aside for the moment the ethical debate over this type of procedure, what the doctors in London achieved gives us a glimpse into the staggering possibilities of medicine in the twenty-first century. Think, for example, of the revolutionary new options available now that the gene for Huntington's chorea has been discovered. Parents may soon be able to decide for themselves if they wish to pass this gene on from one generation to the next.

Designer Babies?

This is, of course, one of the feared outcomes of all that genetic tinkering: that people will be able to designate characteristics in the babies they are about to produce, like hair color, eye color, gender, and brain power. Should an em-

"FRAGILE X": NO KINDER, GENTLER GENES FOR US

*R*ecently, scientists have made an exciting discovery about inherited diseases that could revolutionize the way they are controlled. While studying three genetic diseases of the nervous system, including muscular dystrophy, they learned that the genes actually grow larger with each generation. And the larger the gene, the more severe the disease. They call it the "Fragile X" syndrome.

Remember our botanist monk, Gregor Mendel, who put forth the earliest theories about genetics? He insisted that genes do not get diluted over generations, a finding that fits in neatly with this new discovery. In fact, in some cases the genes can strengthen. This could help explain why inherited cancers, heart diseases, and some other illnesses tend to hit each generation at a younger age.

These extraordinary findings could also explain why some diseases seem to run in families, but in a hit-or-miss pattern. Stronger, nastier genes can surface at any time with a vengeance.

bryo be destroyed, for example, if it isn't the right sex? If it is determined that an embryo has a gene that predisposes it to a certain form of heart disease that may develop forty years later, should it not be allowed to experience the youthful decades of life?

These are not questions out of a science fiction novel. These are very real dilemmas that will soon torment us in our modern medical climate. For now, gene alterations are not passed on to offspring, but the overall role that genetic modifications will play in the evolutionary process has yet to be determined.

Still, as a parent who wonders what insidious genes my son has inherited that might threaten his life, I am thankful scientists are seeking answers to the technical questions of our genetic lives. The ethical debate should thrive alongside the research, and as a society we must put the appropriate restraints on the use of this technology.

No Clones, Please

Remember the provocative but unproven tabloid headlines a few years back about an ego-tistical billionaire creating his own clone in secrecy with the help of a mad scientist? I hope that as researchers learn more about the mystery of genetic messages, the ultimate goal will be to help save lives and to spare children and adults the agony of debilitating disease. The goal should not be to eliminate the mystery of our bodies to the point we are creating life according to some aesthetic whim.

In the meantime, make no mistake about it: The genetic revolution is here. If research continues at its current pace, some medical experts expect to see gene-therapy centers set up all over the country in the not-too-distant future. While such treatments are not without controversy, medical science so far continues its research under strict ethical guidelines.

Can You Inherit Cancer?

In the introduction to this book, you read about my family's personal medical saga. On pages 58–59 you will see our medical family tree, compiled over a period of years with the help of my sisters.

If you examine this tree, you can see that my

GENETIC OR ENVIRONMENTAL? A DINOSAUR GIVES US THE ANSWER.

*T*here is actually something to be learned about genes and disease from dinosaurs, well beyond the provocative premise put forth in Jurassic Park. A couple of years ago, a physician was visiting the Earth Science Museum at Brigham Young University and noticed that one of the dinosaur skeletons had a bone with an odd deformity. It resembled a cauliflower-shaped indentation about the size of a softball.

The bone has since been studied by paleon-tologists, orthopedists, and other doctors, and many of them believe it was nothing more than chrondosarcoma, a form of bone cancer.

Wade Miller, Ph.D., a paleontologist at BYU, estimates the bone to be 136 million years old. That's a good argument that cancer has been around a lot longer in nature than all the toxic elements we believe cause it. After all, there is no known record of dinosaurs smoking, breathing asbestos, or eating the wrong food additives.

own cancer was in the cecum, in the right portion of the colon, or large intestine. This is not a common place for a tumor (most colon tumors are on the left side), which makes the influence of my family's medical history more interesting. Look at my family tree two generations back to my paternal grandfather and see that he, too, had a tumor in the cecum, which killed him at a young age.

Dr. Henry Lynch of the Hereditary Cancer Institute at Creighton University in Omaha has examined our family history on paper and in the laboratory. He says that the cancer in the cecum is sometimes an inherited cancer. Because our family tree specified the location of my grandfather's tumor, it signaled potential trouble. That is why some doctors urged us to get an exam of the entire colon, rather than the more common partial exam. That is the only reason my cancer was caught so early. I should point out that at least one specialist we consulted did not think the full exam was necessary. If I had followed his advice, I'd likely be dead now.

Dr. Lynch says that anywhere from 5 to 10 percent of all cancers are believed to be hereditary, triggered by a specific gene. This accounts for more than one hundred thousand cancer cases each year in the United States alone. In my family, we have what has been dubbed the "Lynch syndrome," a pattern of related cancers that are passed by bad genes traveling through generations. (If you look at my medical family tree, you'll see that my cousin Barb and her father were both hit with pancreatic cancer at the same age. Pancreatic cancer *may* be related to the Lynch syndrome.)

But many other cancers are now considered to be familial, tending to run in families but without seeming to have a direct genetic pattern. In the case of breast cancer, for example, 9 percent of cases are believed to be hereditary, while 25 percent are believed to be familial. A woman with a hereditary thread might have a mother and a sister with the disease. A more common thread would be familial—say, a grandmother and an aunt with breast cancer. I will look at cancer and genetics in greater detail later in this chapter, in Your Own Medical Family Tree Workbook.

Can You Inherit Heart Disease?

The genetic factors in heart disease are also being researched with accelerating speed. A recent study at the University of Utah looked at almost one hundred thousand families and found that individuals with a family history of heart disease had a 5 to 10 percent greater risk of having heart disease themselves. The same study also found that in more than 75 percent of those high-risk families, environmental factors, like smoking or high cholesterol levels, were also present.

But because heredity can influence how the body processes cholesterol, and possibly even provide a predisposition to the habit of smoking cigarettes itself, it is nearly impossible to separate genetic inheritance from environment when assessing your risk of heart disease. There will be more on heart disease in a special section of Your Own Medical Family Tree Workbook.

How Do I Make a Medical Family Tree?

Once you have done some basic genealogy, you are ready to add medical details. In fact, you might have already stumbled onto some useful medical facts.

The next pages provide you with Your Own Medical Family Tree Workbook. No one can get complete details on every ancestor. But the workbook will help you find as much information as possible, and tell you how to analyze it.

WHAT YOU NEED TO KNOW ABOUT GENETIC TESTING

A recent poll by the March of Dimes showed that 68 percent of Americans know "relatively little" or "almost nothing" about genetic testing. But in the same survey, 72 percent said they would take genetic tests to determine if they or their children were at risk for a serious disease. (A Time magazine/CNN poll put the figure at closer to 50 percent.)

By the middle of the next century, there could well be a low-cost comprehensive genetic test available that would predict your risk for a number of deadly diseases. But in the meantime, only those already known to be at risk can be considered for testing. There is only one way to know you are at risk: research your medical family tree.

Genetic Tests Available

Huntington's disease
Cystic fibrosis
Tay-Sachs disease
Sickle-cell anemia
Down's syndrome
Amyotrophic lateral sclerosis
   (Lou Gehrig's disease)
Hemophilia
Gaucher's disease
   (a chronic enzyme deficiency)
Familial polyposis of the colon
   (leads to cancer)

Tests in Development

Familial colon cancer (may include some
   ovarian and uterine cancers)
Neurofibromatosis type 2 (tumors of the
   auditory nerves and tissues)
Kidney cancer
Breast cancer

Genes Almost Isolated

Alzheimer's disease

HEALTH INSURANCE

B ecause genetic testing will be possible long before guaranteed cures, we should all be careful about who gets this personal information, and how it is used. A Time magazine/CNN poll published in 1994 showed that the public was overwhelmingly against allowing employers to use genetic tests to determine whom to hire. But a recent study by the National Academy of Sciences found that Americans were already losing jobs and health insurance because of information uncovered in genetic screens.

So far, only eight states have laws to protect us from these abuses. As state legislatures and Congress consider new laws (in the midst of swirling debate over health insurance in general), you should proceed cautiously. If, after making your medical family tree, you discover you are at risk for a particular illness, you might consider paying cash for a genetic screen without going through your insurance company. Although this could be very expensive, it may be possible to negotiate a payment plan with the laboratory. If a genetic screen determines that you have a familial gene, you may have to let your insurance company know the details so follow-up care can be reimbursed.

AUSTRALIA: SUNNY LABORATORY FOR DEADLY INHERITED SKIN CANCER

There has been much talk about the thinning of the protective ozone layer in the atmosphere and the alarming leap in the number of skin cancers in the United States. The deadliest of those cancers—melanoma—stirs up the nature versus nurture pot in a spicy way.

At Sydney University in Australia, the site of the world's largest human melanoma genetics study, researchers suspect it is a combination of sun and genetics that makes up the sinister brew of damage and disease. If current trends continue, it will soon kill one in one hundred Australians.

This horrific statistic means that the incident of melanoma in Australia has doubled in the past seven years, a rate of growth far beyond normal. One could argue this is environmental—that people are not taking care to protect themselves under an increasingly invasive sun in a hot climate. But researchers in Sydney noticed that some families tend to have more melanoma cases than others, and in 8 percent of those families, the likelihood of developing the disease is almost 100 percent. Does this mean it is due to an inherited gene, or to a careless lifestyle in certain families?

The researchers now believe that it is a combination of both. That some people have defects in the way their bodies repair damage from the sun's ultraviolet radiation. This important research could result in a test to determine who carries the defective gene.

There is worldwide support for the theory that melanoma has a strong genetic factor. Scientists from the National Cancer Institute's epidemiology branch have found a physical trait that is found in people with melanoma: irregular-shaped moles called dysplastic nevus syndrome. The lesions are inherited, and doctors now know they frequently turn malignant. Families with this syndrome are urged to get the moles removed before they become life-threatening.

MIXED CULTURES?

Did any of your relatives marry someone from a nation or culture different from the rest of the family? Did any relative come from racially or ethnically mixed parentage? This is not only interesting and fun to learn about, it can give doctors clues about illnesses that tend to come from certain cultures. You should include such information on your medical family tree.

A classic example of this is found in the bayous of southern Louisiana. An extraordinary number of children there have been hit with what Cajun natives call the "lazy baby" syndrome. In fact, what these children have is Tay-Sachs disease, a tragic inherited disorder that cripples the central nervous system. Most children with Tay-Sachs don't live to see their fifth birthdays.

The illness puzzled doctors for a long time because Tay-Sachs was thought to be found only in descendants of European Jews. Researchers now theorize that a German immigrant brought the gene to the Louisiana area as far back as two hundred years ago.

YOUR OWN MEDICAL FAMILY TREE WORKBOOK

Compiling your medical family history is similar to a regular family tree, except that you need to be more vigilant in obtaining medical information. You will need to focus on blood relatives, but their spouses can be included to determine if a pattern of illness is environmental. For example, suppose your aunt died at a young age of a lung ailment, but never smoked. You might wonder if it was a genetic problem.

But suppose you then learned that her husband (your relative by marriage only) smoked heavily and also died relatively young. Then you can factor in the effect "secondhand smoke" may have had on her health.

Follow the steps below and begin a fascinating trek through your family's health history. Your path to better health will take six steps. You will:

1. Construct the skeleton of your medical family tree.
2. Learn what information you need and how to get it, through death certificates and medical records.

3. Fill in the important medical data on your medical family tree.
4. Learn how to interpret and analyze your medical family tree.
5. Learn details of family heart disease in a special section.
6. Learn how to find the right specialist to help you interpret the tree and possibly offer the necessary diagnostic work.

STEP ONE
Construct the Skeleton of Your Medical Family Tree

Construct your basic "block" family tree. If you have already completed your basic genealogy and the sheet of paper is large enough, you may add medical information directly onto the tree. However, I suggest you use a separate sheet of paper exclusively for your medical family tree. Use large circles for females, large squares for males. Your beginning family tree will look something like our sample on pages 66–67.

Medical Family Tree Skeleton

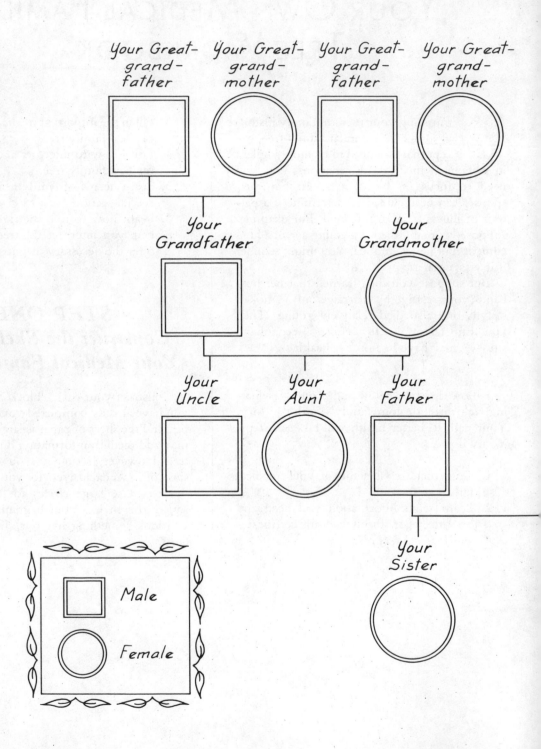

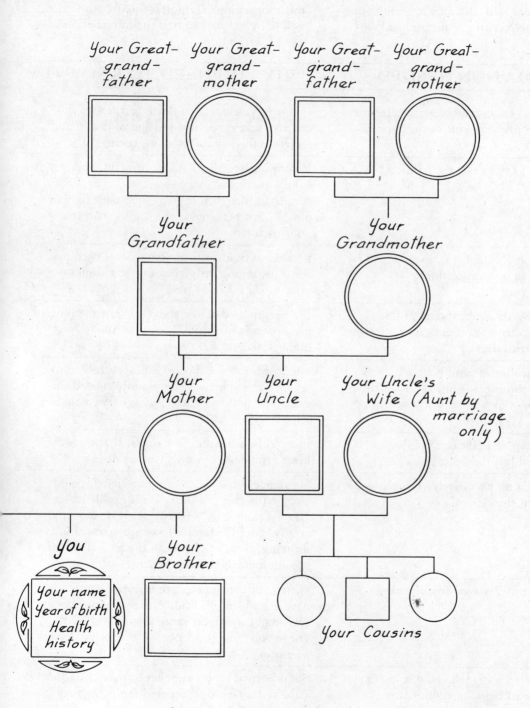

STEP TWO
Gather as Much Medical Information as Possible

The chart below will tell you what you need to know about each relative or ancestor and why the information is important. (After the chart, I will tell you *where* to find the information.)

INFORMATION NEEDED	WHY YOU NEED TO KNOW IT
1. Date of death (Exact date preferred. If you can't get it, then give the year or the approximate year.)	Can help you trace the death certificate, and can also help determine the age of death (and therefore the possibility of a genetic link).
2. Age at death (Try to be as specific as possible.)	If your ancestor died at an unusually young age from a particular illness—one, two, or three decades earlier than most people with the same illness—this becomes a red flag in analyzing your own risk.
3. Cause of death (Note if it is documented by medical records or a death certificate.)	If cause of death was an illness, this becomes the most important piece of information on your medical family tree.
4. If your relative or ancestor died of illness, his or her age at onset (You can often learn this from a death certificate.)	If a person died at age sixty-five but the illness began at age fifty-five, then you might be at higher risk (see #2).
5. Other known illnesses and your relative's age at onset (Again, note if this is documented by medical records or is simply anecdotal information.)	Suppose a relative died of a heart attack at age seventy-five, but was successfully treated for cancer at age fifty. Cancer at age fifty could be a red flag for you.
6. Did relative smoke? (Please note "definitely" or "possibly.")	It could be smoking, not genes, that caused heart problems, cancer, or other diseases.
7. Did relative drink excessively, abuse prescription or illicit drugs?	Substance abuse can run in families. It could also be the cause of other heart problems. A classic example is liver disease: If it runs in a family, does the family have a pattern of heavy drinking? That might mean the liver disease is environmental, and not genetic.
8. Any known miscarriages or stillbirths?	Genetic factors on this are unclear, but if you have a problem with miscarriages, your doctors might treat you more aggressively if they know you have incidences of this in your family history.
9. Do you have relatives who have a history of mental illness or of being institutionalized?	Some mental illness is believed to be hereditary, and a well-documented family history would help health-care professionals keep an

INFORMATION NEEDED	WHY YOU NEED TO KNOW IT
	eye out for early symptoms of mental illness. For more on mental illness and genetics, see Chapter IV, Your Behavioral Family Tree.
10. General physical description • Eye and hair color	This is interesting and fun information that may or may not be significant to your health.
• Height (short, medium, or tall)	For example, some dwarfism is hereditary. If it is in your family, you might want to get genetic counseling before having children. If you don't know an ancestor's skin shade, but do know he had blue eyes and blond hair, chances are he was fair-skinned as well. If he had skin cancer, this could be important information (see below).
• Race and skin color (To designate shade of skin use terms "fair," "medium," or "dark")	Very important in tracking skin cancers. For example, fair-skinned people are more likely to get skin lesions from sun exposure. If you have dark-skinned ancestors with skin cancers, it is more likely to be genetic. However, any family pattern puts you at higher risk. Race is also important in tracking certain illnesses that tend to be seen exclusively in one race. (Sickle-cell anemia, for example, is seen only among African-Americans.)
• Weight ("Very thin," "normal," "overweight," or "obese")	A look at weight patterns on your medical family tree could be very important to your future health. Some obesity is genetic, and you could be forewarned of the dangers.
11. Any unusual physical characteristics? (For example, persistent rash or skin problems, blindness, deafness, early baldness, facial tics.)	These could signal any number of inherited conditions and should be noted on your medical family tree.

Where do I find this information?

1. Oral histories: They are a good beginning, but only a beginning. Talk to as many relatives as possible, especially the oldest ones. Family lore can be fun, but it's not medically reliable. It's interesting to have Uncle Joe tell you his grandma Sadie had a bad heart, but it's not much help to your doctor. Written confirmation that she died of a sudden heart attack at age fifty-six is much better information. A pattern of early heart attacks might mean you have the same predisposition.

2. Death certificates: These are perhaps your most valuable source of information. Death certificates list more than the cause of death. If your ancestor died of an illness, a death certificate will usually list the length of the illness, which lets you know the age of onset (critical in determining your risk of getting that illness).

Death certificates can be fascinating and full of surprises. When I finally got around to sending for my Aunt Bertha's death certificate, it came back with a stunning revelation. The "stomach or colon" cancer that killed her turned out to be carcinoma of the ovary. It was 1942 and such "delicate" cancers weren't discussed much, even among family members. But it showed us that we had ovarian cancers striking young women on both sides of my family, which explains why our generation was hit so hard with the disease.

Death certificates can also give unexpected additional information. It was my grandmother Bird's death certificate that told us her uterine cancer was diagnosed at age fifty-six. That

made her death at age sixty-two more significant. The younger the onset, the more likely it is an inherited disease. Death certificates will also sometimes tell you if there had been recent surgery or other illnesses or complications. And you can learn information that could lead you to valuable medical records.

In summary, here is what you might be able to learn about your ancestors from death certificates:

1. Cause of death
2. Age at death
3. Length of illness

OBESITY: IS IT INHERITED OR ARE YOU JUST EATING TOO MUCH?

The answer to this tortuous question probably falls right in the middle of these two conflicting theories. Studies of twins and adopted children have shown that at least half the problems with obesity are genetically determined.

Identical twins (who have the same genes) are much more alike in body weight and fat distribution than fraternal twins, who share, on average, half the same genes. Other studies have shown that adopted children are much more like their biological parents in weight and fat distribution than the parents who adopt and raise them.

A study at Laval University in Quebec overfed volunteers (twin pairs) by a thousand calories a day. Most sets of twins gained weight at the same pace. Interestingly, some pairs gained a little, some a lot. Similar studies have prompted many researchers to conclude that the body is programmed to stay within a particular weight range. This would explain why dieters who lose weight usually gain it back. One researcher, Dr. Janet Polivy (a psychologist the University of Toronto),

has publicly declared, "It's time we started treating body weight more like height, as a biologically determined trait."

This is not meant to provide careless overeaters with an excuse not to control their eating habits (and thus imperil their health). But if you know the tendency toward being overweight is genetic, you might take diet and nutrition more seriously. As a young person, look at your mother and father and other relatives. Do you see obesity? Then consult a doctor and nutritionist and develop a realistic eating and exercise plan.

There is a flip side to the weight coin. If you aspire to look like an eighteen-year-old supermodel, a look at your parents and other relatives might be a good reality check. Maybe you are programmed to be ten or twenty pounds heavier than those skinny bodies that decorate the fashion magazines. Your body may be sending you a message that it wants those few extra pounds, and as long as you are taking good care of yourself, perhaps you should accept your genetic fate with pleasure.

4. Surgeries related to illness
5. Name of doctor
6. Place of death
7. Usual residence
8. Name of hospital
9. Name of mortician
10. Name and location of cemetery
11. Occupation
12. Marital status
13. Name of spouse
14. Name of ancestor's father
15. Mother's maiden name
16. Other illnesses or medical conditions

How do I get my hands on the right death certificates?

Every state and some countries have an office called something like "Division of Vital Records" or "Bureau of Vital Statistics." For a small fee (usually about $5.00), they will send you a copy of an ancestor's death certificate. It will be an uncertified copy, but that is all you need to properly document medical information (For a complete list of addresses, see Where to Write for Death Certificates on pages 157–64.)

What do I say in the letter?

You will need to write a letter (see sample letter page 77) to the office in your state, explaining why you want a copy, and what your relationship is to the deceased. Because every state will require slightly different information in order to send you a death certificate, it is best to cover all bases. In your request, include as much of the following information as possible:

1. Full name of the deceased relative (including maiden name).
2. Your relationship to the person.
3. Reason for wanting the death certificate.
4. Date of death (year or range of years is acceptable, although you might be charged extra for every year searched).
5. Age at death (approximate, if necessary).
6. County or city where death occurred.
7. Name of spouse of deceased relative.
8. Name of parents of deceased relative (you or an energetic clerk might be able to trace the location of death through the birth certificate and location of birth).
9. Social Security number of deceased (it's not likely you will know this, but if you do, it can help the clerk's search).

NEW TWIST ON ARTHRITIS

*W*ho would have thought that a small group of Pacific islanders would hold the key to a gene that can prevent rheumatoid arthritis?

Researchers at the Auckland Medical School in New Zealand have discovered that Maori and Pacific islanders have a rare gene that makes them less likely to develop the disabling disease.

Their findings illustrate how complicated genetic research can be. It has been known for some time that many people who carry a certain gene are at greater risk for rheumatoid arthritis. Yet the islanders, who get the disease only in rare cases, have a variant of that gene. Those who do develop the crippling form of arthritis have a different variant. It is now up to researchers to focus on the difference between the two.

One possible result: Scientists may learn ways to negate the effects of the arthritis-prone gene. If the gene could be neutralized, sufferers could be treated with gene therapy, and be free of medication, which is often ineffective or loaded with rough side-effects.

3. *Medical Records:* Collecting death certificates for your family will be enough to make a useful medical family tree. But if you see a serious illness or death at a young age, you should at least try to get your hands on that relative's or ancestor's medical records. It might not be easy, but here are some suggested methods:

A. If that relative is still living, try to get the medical records now. Explain to him or her that you would be happy to be the record-keeper in the family, and that all the information will be kept confidential. During serious illness, some family members are in an understandable state of denial and might not want to share records. Others will feel good knowing they can contribute to better health for the rest of the family. (See sample letters on pages 79 and 80.)

B. If a relative does not want to give you medical records, quietly encourage the next-of-kin to keep copies of all records in a safe place. You can ask again at a later time. Encourage the next-of-kin to keep any autopsy records.

C. After a relative has died, you can request records from the doctor if you are next-of-kin. If you are not, gently encourage the next-of-kin to make the request. You can even prepare the letter yourself and ask the next-of-kin to approve and sign it. (See sample letter on page 81.) You will know where to write by looking at the name of the hospital or doctor on the death certificate, and the location of death. The hospital might well still exist, even if the doctor is no longer alive.

D. Some states have strict privacy laws and it can be tough to get medical records, but don't give up easily. The death certificate will usually state the location of the doctor's office and/or the hospital where your relative was treated. The first step is to contact the doctor's office and see what further steps are necessary to obtain the medical records. If the doctor is no longer living, contact the hospital.

E. If the information in your relative's records could have a crucial bearing on your health, you might have to hire a lawyer to help you obtain them. Later in this section we'll discuss how to know if the information is important.

F. If all else fails, one physician I know suggests a "back door" method for obtaining medical records. If you know the name and location of the hospital where your relative was treated (again, this is usually listed on the death certificate), make a "consultation" appointment with a doctor who has privileges at the hospital that keeps the records you need. When you arrive for your appointment, bring a letter from your physician or geneticist explaining your need to have the information. Hopefully, the doctor will at least look up the records to see if they contain details you need to know. If you can't go in person, you might be able to achieve results by mail or over the phone.

G. If you are going several generations back, it is very possible the relative died at home, and there might not be any medical records. I got my hands on my great-grandmother's death certificate, and the cause of death was listed as "Tumor of——." Her age at death was listed as thirty-seven, but the exact type of cancer remains a mystery. Still, the fact she apparently died of cancer at such a young age makes us suspect that our family's history of cancer goes back at least that far (she died in 1885, yet the state of Wisconsin found the death certificate easily).

Sample Death Certificates

There is a wealth of information found on death certificates

"Metastatic Carcinoma"

"Primary carcinoma of colon"

"Primary carcinoma of pancreas"

"weeks"

"months"

Form No. 210—9-41—25M
Original Certificate of DEATH

WISCONSIN STATE BOARD OF HEALTH
Bureau of Vital Statistics

OCT 9 1942

Local Registrar's No. ____

1. PLACE OF DEATH:

(a) County ___Dane___

(b) Township ___Westport___
or
City or Village ____

(c) Name of hospital
or institution ____

2. USUAL RESIDENCE OF DECEASED:

(a) State ___Wisconsin___ (b) County ___Dane___

(c) Township ___Westport___
or   If rural give township
City or Village ____

(d) Street No. ____

(e) If foreign born, how long in U. S. A.? ____

3. (a) Full Name ___Bertha Moore___

3. (b) If veteran,
name war ____

3. (c) Social Security
No. ___None___

4. Sex ___F___ | 5. Color or race ___W___ | 6. (a) Single, widowed, married, divorced ___Married___

6. (b) Name of husband or wife
___Leslie R. Moore___

6. (c) Age of husband or wife if
alive ___53___ years.

7. Birth date of deceased ___May___ ___23___ ___1910___
(Month) (Day) (Year)

8. AGE: Years ___32___ | Months ___2___ | Days ___26___ | If less than one day hr. ___ min. ___

9. Birthplace ___Milwaukee___ ___Wisconsin___
(City, town, or county) (State or foreign country)

10. Occupation and industry or business ___Phone operator___

Father { 11. Name ___E. Krause___
{ 12. Birthplace ___Not known___
(City, town, or county) (State or foreign country)

Mother { 13. Maiden name ___Martha Bochlke___
{ 14. Birthplace ___Milwaukee, Wisconsin___
(City, town, or county) (State or foreign country)

15. (a) Informant ___Leslie R. Moore___
(b) Address ___Mendota, Wisconsin___

16. (a) ___Burial___ (b) Date thereof ___8-22-42___
(Burial, cremation or other)   (Mo.)(Da.)(Yr.)

(c) Place: burial or cremation ___Roselawn___

17. (a) Signature of funeral director ___A.A. Frautschi___
(b) Address ___Madison, Wisconsin___

18. (a) ___Sept 8 1942___ (b) ____
(Date received local registrar)   (Registrar's signature)

(c) ___8/20/42___ (d) ____
(Date received sub-registrar)   (Sub-registrar's signature)

MEDICAL CERTIFICATION ___49a___

19. Date of death: Month ___8___ Day ___18___ Year ___42___

20. I hereby certify that I attended the deceased from ___3-9___ ___1942___
to ___8-18___, 1942. I last saw her alive on ___8-2___, 1942
and that death occurred on the date stated above at ____ M.

Immediate cause of death ____

Due to ____

Duration ___6 mn___

Other conditions ____
Include pregnancy within 3 months of death

Name of operation ____   Date ___3-9-42___

Major findings
Of operation ____

Physician
Underline the
cause to which
death should
be charged
statistically.

Of autopsy ____

**UNCERTIFIED
NOT VALID FOR
IDENTIFICATION PURPOSES**

21. If death was due to external causes, fill in the following:

(a) Accident, suicide or homicide ____   (b) Date ____

(c) Where did injury occur ____
(City, village or township, county and state)

(d) Did injury occur in or about home, on farm, in industrial place,
in public place? ____   While at work? ____
(Specify type of place)

(e) Means of injury ____
(Fall? Auto? Machinery? etc.)

22. Signature ____ (M. D. or other)
Address ___Madison, Wisconsin___   Date signed ___8-19-42___

She had surgery
six months
before her death
which indicates
an accurate
diagnosis

MARYLAND STATE DEPARTMENT OF HEALTH
2411 N. Charles St., Baltimore

CERTIFICATE OF DEATH

14328

Reg. Dist. No. *246*

1. PLACE OF DEATH:
County *Prince George*
City or town *Cheverly*
(If outside city or town limits, write RURAL and give nearest town)
How long in above place of death?
Hospital, institution, or street address where death occurred:

How long in hospital or institution?

2. USUAL RESIDENCE (HOME) OF DECEASED
(For newborn infants give residence of mother)
State *Maryland* County *Prince George*
City or town *Cheverly*
(If outside city or town limits, write RURAL and give nearest town)
Street No. *3001- Crest Ave*
(If rural, give LOCATION)
2.(a) If veteran, name war

3. (a) FULL NAME *Bird Hitchock Fraser*

3. (b) Social Security Number

4. Sex *Female* **5. Color or race** *White* **6.(a) Single, married, widowed, or divorced** *Married*

MEDICAL CERTIFICATION

6.(b) Name of husband or wife *Curther Fraser*

20. DATE OF DEATH *12 - 6* 19 *42*, at *10:45* M

7. Birth date of deceased (mo., day, yr.) *June 6th 1880*
6.(c) If alive, give age *71* years

21. I CERTIFY that death occurred on the date above stated; that I attended deceased from *9-14* 19 *42*, to *12 - 6* 19 *42*
and that I last saw her alive on *12 - 6* 19 *42*

8. AGE: Years *62* Months *6* Days *0* If less than one day — hrs. — min.

Immediate cause of death *Carcinoma of body of uterus with extensive metastases*

DURATION *5 yrs*

9. Birthplace *West Salem Wisc.*
(Town, county, and state)

Due to

10. Usual occupation

Due to

11. Industry or business

Other conditions

FATHER 12. Name *Philip Hitchock*
13. Birthplace *Ohio*

(Include pregnancy within 8 months of death)

MOTHER 14. Maiden name *Ida Slater*
15. Birthplace *Ohio*

Major findings of operations............................Date of op.

16. Informant *Curther Fraser*
Address *3001- Crest Ave. Cheverly*

Autopsy results.
PHYSICIAN: Please underline the cause to which death should be charged statistically.

17. *(Burial, cremation, or removal. Which?)* Date thereof *12 - 9 1942*
(month) (day) (year)
Cemetery or crematory *Hancock*
Location *Wisconsin*

22. VIOLENCE: If death was due to external causes, fill in the following:
Accident, suicide, or homicide............................Date of.....
Where did injury occur?
(City or town) (County) (State)
Injured at home, farm, industry, public place (where?)
Means of injury Injured at work?

18. Funeral director *Wm J Galley*
Address *3200- R.J Ave Mt Rainier Md.*
Mr Harry Galley

23. SIGNATURE *W Burman* M.D.
M. D. or other
Address *Mt. Rainier Md* Date signed *12-7-42*

19. *12-9-42* 19
(Date rec'd by registrar) Registrar

"Carcinoma of body
of uterus with
extensive metastases"

"This shows she was
much younger
when diagnosed"

CERTIFICATE OF DEATH

DECEDENT—NAME	First	Middle	Last	SEX	DATE OF DEATH (Mo. Day, Year)
	DELPHINE	ANTOINETTE	KROESEN	Female	February 1, 1984

RACE—(e.g. White, Black, American Indian, etc.) (Specify)	AGE—Last Birthday (Years)	UNDER 1 YEAR Mos. Days	UNDER 1 DAY Hours Mins.	DATE OF BIRTH (Mo. Day, Yr.)	COUNTY OF DEATH
White	87			April 16, 1896	Cuyahoga

CITY, VILLAGE OR LOCATION OF DEATH	HOSPITAL OR OTHER INSTITUTION—Name (If not in either, give street and number)	IF HOSP OR INST INDICATE DOA, OP/Emer Rm, Inpatient (Specify)
Middleburg Heights	Southwest General Hospital	Inpatient

STATE OF BIRTH (If not in U.S.A. name country)	CITIZEN OF WHAT COUNTRY	ORIGIN OR DESCENT (Italian, Mexican, German, English, Cuban, Puerto Rican, etc.) (Specify)	SOCIAL SECURITY NUMBER
Ohio	USA	American	270-10-8675

WAS DECEASED EVER IN U.S. ARMED FORCES? (Yes, no, or unknown)	MARRIED, NEVER MARRIED, WIDOWED, DIVORCED (Specify)	SURVIVING SPOUSE (If wife, give maiden name)
No	Never Married	

USUAL OCCUPATION (Give kind of work done during most of working life, even if retired)	KIND OF BUSINESS OR INDUSTRY
Buyer	Bailey Co. Dept. Stores

RESIDENCE—STATE	COUNTY	CITY, VILLAGE OR LOCATION	STREET AND NUMBER	INSIDE CITY LIMITS (Specify Yes or No)
Ohio	Cuyahoga	Olmsted Falls	8801 Lindberg Blvd.	Yes

FATHER—NAME			MOTHER—MAIDEN NAME		
John	G.	Kroesen	Mary	Helen	Blumena

INFORMANT—NAME	MAILING	(CITY OR TOWN) (STATE) (ZIP)
James Paul Kroesen	8	Olmsted Falls, Ohio 44138

"Acute Inferolateral Myocardial Infarction"

PART I.	DEATH WAS CAUSED BY: [ENTER ... AND (c)]	APPROXIMATE INTERVAL BETWEEN ONSET AND DEATH
18. IMMEDIATE CAUSE	(a) *Acute Inferolateral Myocardial Infarction* DUE TO, OR AS A CONSEQUENCE OF:	8 days
	(b) *Hypertensive & Arteriosclerotic Heart Disease* DUE TO, OR AS A CONSEQUENCE OF:	15—20 years
	(c)	

PART II. OTHER SIGNIFICANT CONDITIONS: Conditions contributing to death but not related to cause given in Part I	AUTOPSY (Yes or no)	WAS CASE REFERRED TO CORONER (Yes or No)
Early maturity onset Diabetes Mellitus; Diverticulitis c abscess formation	No	

"Early maturity onset Diabetes Mellitus"

"Diverticulitis with abscess formation"

"Hypertension and Arteriosclerotic Heart Disease"

ACC., SUICIDE, HOM., UNDET. OR PENDING INQUEST (Specify)	DATE OF INJURY (Month, Day, Year)	HOUR	HOW INJURY OCCURRED (Enter nature of injury in Part I or Part II, item 18)
20a.			
20b. INJURY AT WORK (Specify yes or no)			
20c.			

To be Completed by ATTENDING PHYSICIAN Only		To be Co...
21a. To the best of my knowledge, death occurred at the time, date and place and due to the cause(s) stated. (Signature and Title) *Myron J. Welty, M.D.*	22a. On the basis of examination and/or ... and place and due to the cause(s) stated. (Signature and Title)	
21b. DATE SIGNED (Mo. Day, Year) 2-2-84	21c. HOUR OF DEATH 2:20 A. M	22b. DATE SIGNED (Mo. Day, Year)
		22c. HOUR OF DEATH M
		22d. PRONOUNCED DEAD (Mo. Day, Year) On	PRONOUNCED DEAD (Hour) AT M

NAME AND ADDRESS OF CERTIFIER (PHYSICIAN OR CORONER) (Type or Print)	(Street or R.F.D. no., city or village, state, zip)
23 *226 Front Street, Berea, Ohio 44017*	

BURIAL, CREMATION, OTHER (Specify)	DATE	NAME OF CEMETERY OR CREMATORY	LOCATION (City, village, or county) (State)
24a. Burial	24b. Feb. 4, 1984	24c. St. Mary of the Falls	24d. Olmsted Falls, Ohio

NAME OF EMBALMER	(LIC. No.)	FUNERAL DIRECTOR'S SIGNATURE	(LIC. No.)
25 Roger F. Baker	6315-A	26 *Richard A. Baker*	4771

FUNERAL FIRM AND ADDRESS	(STREET NO.)	(CITY)	(STATE)	(ZIP)
27 Baker Funeral Home	206 Front Street	Berea, Ohio	44017	

DATE REC'D FEB 2 1984	REGISTRAR'S SIGNATURE *E. C. Fern*	DATE PERMIT ISSUED FEB 2 1984	SIGNATURE OF PERSON ISSUING PERMIT *Same*

I HEREBY CERTIFY THAT THE ABOVE IS AN EXACT
COPY OF THE RECORD WHICH IS ON FILE IN THE
DEPARTMENT OF HEALTH, CLEVELAND, OHIO.
WITNESS MY HAND AND SEAL AS LOCAL REGISTRAR
OF VITAL STATISTICS.

E. C. Fern

FEB 02 1984
REGISTRAR

Sample Letter:

How to send for a death certificate

Lawrence Smith
Springlake Drive
Madison, WI 53701
(608)555-1116

5/9/93

The Office of the State Registrar
304 S Street
P.O. Box 730241
Sacramento, CA 95814-0241

To the Office of the State Registrar:

I represent the Harold Smith family of Madison, Wisconsin. We are researching the possibility of hereditary disease in our extended family and would like a copy of a death certificate for Joanne Smith Williams, my grandmother on my father's side.

We believe she died in the city of Oakland, California, around 1941 at the age of fifty-six. Her husband's name was Eugene Lawrence Williams, who is also deceased. I do not know the name of the funeral director who handled her remains.

I have enclosed a check for $8.00. If you are unable to find the death certificate for Joanne Smith Williams and need more payment to search additional years, please let me know at the above address.

Thank you very much for this important information.

Sincerely,

(Signature)

Lawrence Smith

Letter for Your Use:

You may remove the sample letter below from this book, photocopy it, and fill in the blanks.
If you do not know all the information, simply write "not known" in the blank.

My Name _____
My Address _____
Daytime phone _____

Date _____

The Office of _____
Address _____

               _____
               _____

To Whom It May Concern:

    I represent the _____ family of _____ .
We are researching the possibility of hereditary disease in our
extended family and would like a copy of the death certificate
for_____, my_____ .
    We believe _____ died in the city of
_____ around _____ at the age of
_____. The remains were handled by_____.
    I have enclosed a check in the amount of $_____.
If you are unable to find the death·certificate for
_____ and need additional payment to search
additional years, please, let me know at the above address.
    Thank you very much for this important information.

                                   Sincerely,

                                   Signature: _____

                                   Printed name: _____

Sample Letter:

Asking the family for medical information

```
                              Your Name
                              Your Address
                              Your Home Phone and Daytime Phone

                              Date


Dear_____  ,


     Greetings to all in the_____ extended clan. I
hope you can help me with an important project.
     I am currently researching information that could be vital
to the health of each one of us, especially to our children and
grandchildren. I am attempting to put together a ''medical''
family tree that will record illnesses and causes of death for
as many generations back as possible.
     New scientific research has shown that many, many illnesses
and behavioral patterns could have a hereditary, or genetic,
link. If we know the risk in advance, our doctors can help us
get the right check-ups and tests.
     I am enclosing a copy of our family tree, with as much
information as I have. Would each of you help me fill in the
blanks and make corrections? Any extra information or tidbits
about the lifestyle, health habits, or profession of each
relative would be useful. We need to distinguish environmental
causes from possible hereditary ones. For example, we need to
know if each relative smoked or drank heavily, etc.
     I how that for some of us sharing this information could
bring back painful memories. But once I have the most accurate
information possible, I will seek the advice of an expert in
hereditary diseases. I will be happy to share with each of you
what I have learned. This literally could save lives in our
family.
     Please contact me if you have any questions!


                              With love to all,


                              Your name
```

Sample Letter:

Asking an ill relative for medical records

Your Name
Your Address
Your Phone Number

Date

Dear_____ ,

    I hope this letter finds you feeling as lively and well as possible—and I hope the doctors haven't been too rough on you! Every day I send good thoughts and energy your way.

    As you may know, I am somewhat of a family librarian when it comes to keeping track of medical problems. New research has shown that many, many ailments can have a genetic link, or could have been caused by a combination of environmental and hereditary problems.

    I am trying to keep a file of medical records so future generations can continue to build our medical family tree. Would it be an inconvenience to ask you for copies of your medical records? It is easiest to get them from you directly. All you have to do is ask your doctor for extra copies. Maybe it can be done by those interns and residents who follow your case along with your primary physician. Or I would be happy to make copies for you.

    I promise to keep all the records confidential, and not share the details with other family members. From time to time I'll take our family records to an expert in hereditary diseases, and I'll share with the rest of the family the general nature of what I have learned. Knowing our risks in advance means we can get the right kind of check-ups and tests.

    This is a simple gift you can give to the children of our family, and I can assure you I will take good care of all the records.

    Take good care of yourself, and call me with any questions! Anytime!

Thinking of you always,

Your Name

Sample Letter:

How to send for medical records

```
                                    Your Name
                                    Your Address
                                    Your Phone Number

                                    Date


Dr. John Doe
Main Street
Journeytown, MA 02190

Dear Dr. Doe:

    I represent the family of (name) of (city, state). We
believe he was your patient from (years). He died of cancer in
(year) at the (name of hospital). (ancestor's name) was my
father's uncle. My father is deceased and, as far as I know, I
am _____'s closest living relative.
    Our family physician suggested that medical records could
answer some vital questions as we research the possibility of
hereditary disease in our extended family. We are compiling
records to have them analyzed by an expert in genetic disease.
    Please send me copies of (ancestor's name) medical records,
or advise me how to arrange for copies. Please understand that
this information could be critical to all of us in the (family
name) family, especially to our children.
    Thank you for the time this might involve. Please contact me
at the above phone number and address if you have any questions.

                                    Sincerely,



                                    Your name
```

STEP THREE
Fill in the Information on Your Medical Family Tree

The chart on the next page is an enlarged sample of how to organize the information under each relative's name. The format for this chart will be a circle (if your relative is female) or a square (if your relative is a male).

Adoptees may want to know more about their biological family because of the number of illnesses that do have a genetic component. Awareness of a biological tree is key to seeking early detection of potentially life-threatening diseases. (It may also help if ever an organ transplant is needed and the most likely donor candidates are blood relatives.) In addition, adoptees may want to be knowledgeable about their relatives' medical histories so they can make informed decisions about planning their own families.

There are many emotional issues that go into

WHAT IF YOU'RE ADOPTED?

*M*y friend Sally Henderson, who was adopted at birth, had always known her biological mother died at a young age. But the cause was a mystery. That was, until the age of twenty-eight, when Sally was diagnosed with a precancerous condition in her cervix. At the urging of her doctor, she began to search for her genetic history.

She wrote to the adoption agency in Minnesota that had placed her and included a note from her doctor. The agency told her how to petition a local judge to have her adoption records opened. The judge did so, and she learned her mother had died of breast cancer when she was only forty-four years old. Sally was not given the identity of her birth mother, but was given her medical history.

Sally began active breast-cancer screening, which also included screenings for gynecological cancers. Her vigilance paid off. At age forty-one she was diagnosed as having an early-stage cancer in her uterus, and she has since been successfully treated.

The connection between breast and ovarian cancer is well established, but the connection between breast and uterine cancer is unclear. But because both cancers involve the hormone estrogen, and because doctors knew her family history, their aggressive approach saved Sally's life.

The story doesn't end there. Sally eventually learned about two brothers she never knew she had. After her cancer diagnosis, she decided she had to meet them. They invited her to a family reunion, where dozens of her blood relatives gathered to meet their long-lost kin. "When they first saw me," she told me, "I could hear them gasp. I'm the same age now as my mother was when she died. They say I look exactly like her."

Ironically, Sally spent much of that reunion sharing medical tales with a first cousin who had just had a double mastectomy at age forty-four, the same age at which Sally's mother died of breast cancer.

Happily, Sally is doing well and is grateful she can warn her newly found relatives of the risks they face. This story shows that adoptees who are successful in searching for their biological parents should also seek medical information.

the decision to search for one's birth parents: The need to learn more about your medical past is certainly one of them. (Of course, for many adoptees it's impossible to trace their biological history.) If your genetic heritage remains a puzzle, you can at least be the one who starts the valuable process of record-keeping so your children and grandchildren will have a well-nurtured family tree.

For guidance on how to begin an adoption search, write the Adoptees Liberty Movement Association (ALMA):

ALMA
Post Office Box 154
Washington Bridge Station
New York, NY 10033

NAME _____

OCCUPATION _____

CAUSE OF DEATH _____

AGE _____ *ONSET* _____

SMOKER/DRINKER? _____

OTHER HEALTH HISTORY _____

_____

_____

PHYSICAL DESCRIPTION _____

_____

OTHER COMMENTS _____

_____

_____

◯ = **FEMALE**   ☐ = **MALE**

STEP FOUR
Interpret and Analyze Your Medical Family Tree

First, keep in mind the difference between first- and second-degree relatives. First-degree relatives share up to half the same genes. They would be brothers, sisters, parents, or children. Second-degree relatives share one-fourth of the same genes. These would be aunts, uncles, and grandparents. (For greater clarification, refer to the tree chart in Chapter I on page 17.)

Finding a pattern of illness doesn't necessarily mean you are at any greater risk. But it is something your doctor should know. Here's how to tell if you need to go beyond your family doctor and consult a specialist:

- Did two or more relatives have the same disease?
- Did a young first- or second-degree relative have an illness usually associated with older people (for example, cancer or heart disease at age thirty, forty, or fifty)?

Red Flag

See a specialist right away if you discover the following:
- Two first-degree relatives with the same cancer (breast, uterine, ovarian, and colon should be considered the "same").
- One first-degree relative under the age of fifty with cancer or serious heart disease.

Cancer terms:

Cancer terms found on death certificates and medical records come in several categories:
1. General terms
   - carcinoma
   - tumor

COMMON INHERITED CANCERS

At least 100,000 cancer cases a year are believed to be hereditary.

BREAST: 180,000 new cases a year; 5 to 10 percent directly hereditary: Family pattern seen in 25 percent of cases.

OVARIAN: 20,000 new cases a year: Family pattern seen in 10 percent of cases.

COLORECTAL: 156,000 new cases a year: Family pattern seen in 10 percent of cases.

MELANOMA: 30,000 new cases a year: Family pattern seen in 10 percent of cases.

PANCREATIC: 30,000 new cases a year: Family pattern seen in at least 5 percent of cases.

LUNG: 168,000 new cases a year: Because of smoking, air pollution, and other environmental factors, it is unknown what percentage comes directly from "bad genes."

ENDOMETRIAL (lining of the uterus): 35,000 new cases a year: Unknown percentage runs in families. Cervical cancer is not known to be genetic.

PROSTATE: 132,000 new cases a year. There seems to be some familial association, but it could be connected more to high-fat diets than to genes.

Probable Family Connection: Cancer of the kidney and leukemia. Researchers also suspect that there may be a link between certain genetic disorders and leukemia.

- malignancy: indicates existence of cancer
- metastases: indicates spread of cancer

2. Words that end in "oma"
   Examples—
   - lymphoma: cancer of the lymph nodes
   - osteosarcoma: cancer of the bone
   - multiple myeloma: abnormal plasma cells that destroy bones

3. Leukemias (blood cancers)
   Examples—
   - lymphocytic leukemia
   - myeloid leukemia

4. Organ cancers
   The majority of cancers striking major organs are simply called by the name of the diseased organ, such as "kidney cancer," "stomach cancer," or "lung cancer."

5. Cancers named after researchers. If you can't identify the type of disease, write the full name right on the family tree. A doctor can identify it for you.
   Examples—
   - Hodgkin's disease: a form of lymphoma
   - Bowen's disease: a form of skin cancer

CANCER: GET SPECIFICS!

*T*here are important facts to know about certain illnesses. Some information is always better than none, but there are reasons to dig beyond a simple mention of "cancer," or even "breast cancer." You can use a death certificate or medical records to get additional information. You can also obtain more material from oral histories, but remember that such details only provide possible clues. Medical documentation is always your best bet.

Look for answers to these questions about specific cancers:

BREAST: Was illness "unilateral" (one breast) or "bilateral" (both breasts)? Bilateral cancer tends to be more genetic, and if you find this on your family tree, you should immediately inform your doctor.

SKIN: Was it "melanoma" (the most deadly and believed to be the most genetic), "basal cell," or "squamous cell"? If you have any of these on your family tree, you should see a dermatologist (skin doctor) regularly and get advice on how to protect your skin.

OVARIAN: Did the disease start outside the ovary (it happens in 10 percent of the cases). That could indicate a chance that it is genetic. Also, what was the "stage" and "grade" of the disease? (These terms are used to describe the degree and severity of the disease.) A higher stage or grade means a greater chance it is genetic.

COLORECTAL: Where was the tumor located? Right side, top, or left side? In the rectum? (Tumors on the right side or in the cecum could indicate a bad gene and might increase your own risk.) Did relative have lots of benign polyps (a condition known as "polyposis") discovered as well? Polyposis usually leads to cancer, and is very genetic. If this is on your family tree, you need to be checked more frequently.

OTHER CANCERS: In cases of cancers with tumors, try to determine the exact location of tumor. For any cancer, can you find out what the first symptoms were? There's no guarantee you would have the same symptoms, but it's useful information that might get you to the doctor more quickly.

BREAST CANCER BREAKTHROUGH

*I*t has been known for some time that breast cancer runs in families. The how and why is complicated, but soon we will have effective control over many inherited breast cancers.

What has been a distant dream for women threatened with this terrible disease is about to burst into real life. By the time this book is published, researchers at several cancer centers hope to have actually identified the gene for some genetic breast cancers. This breakthrough could dramatically alter the lives of women at risk, and give doctors a clear target gene to attack. Soon to follow will be a test so women will know if they carry the gene.

Women who have two first-degree relatives with breast cancer (a sister and mother, for example) carry a horrifying 50 percent risk. If they can determine they don't carry the gene, their risk will drop to about 10 percent—about the same as women who don't have breast cancer in their family history. Either way, discovery of the gene will help women and their doctors make choices about how to proceed with medical check-ups.

Breast cancer is a disease that will hit one in nine women in their lifetime, a statistic that has grown because women with strong family histories of breast cancer are included. Discovery of the gene will change the whole face of the disease and is a godsend to women at risk.

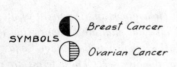

How Breast Cancer Can Look on a Family Tree

This is a copy of a medical family tree of a family studied at Cedars Sinai Medical Center in Beverly Hills, California. It shows a breast/ovarian cancer syndrome. NOTE HOW IT CAN BE PASSED THROUGH A FATHER.

A slash indicates the person is deceased. Note that one woman had both cancers. Women with either breast or ovarian cancer in their family should know they could be at high risk for both.

See pages 166–67 for places to contact for more information.

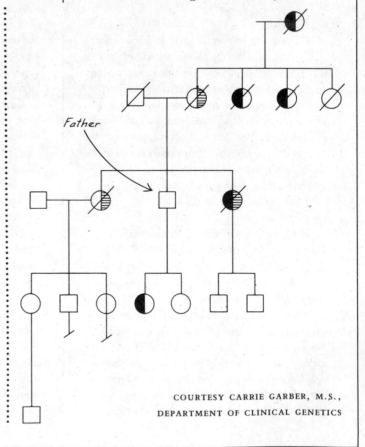

COURTESY CARRIE GARBER, M.S.,
DEPARTMENT OF CLINICAL GENETICS

STEP FIVE
How Can I Tell if My Family's Heart Disease Is Putting Me at Risk?

Because everyone has heart attacks and heart disease in the family, it is easy to overlook what might be a genetic pattern. After all, dying of "old age" is essentially dying of heart failure.

Heart failure can also be the end result of another illness. My father battled prostate cancer for years. When the cancer finally invaded his spine, he became terribly weak and his heart just stopped beating. The coroner listed his death as "heart failure" on the death certificate, although cancer was what took its toll on his body and heart.

Heart disease as a primary cause of death is still the biggest killer in the United States. Seventy million Americans currently have some form of heart or cardiovascular disease. But if you think it's just a problem for "old folks,"

think again. Nearly two hundred thousand of those who die from it every year are under sixty-five. To look at it another way: Of all the heart attacks recorded every year in this country, 43 percent hit people under sixty-five years of age. Every year in this country, twenty-five thousand Americans under the age of forty have heart attacks. And someone dies from cardiovascular disease every thirty-four seconds.

The good news is that death rates from heart disease are declining, partly because of advanced medical treatment and partly because people are becoming more aware of their family histories and taking better care of themselves. In fact, in the next decade, cancer is expected to surpass heart disease as the nation's leading killer.

DIABETES: A HEARTFELT MATTER

*A*bout 5 percent of Americans are diabetic. Diabetics do not produce enough insulin from their pancreas, which means that the level of glucose in their blood is excessively high. Seventy-five percent of diabetics die from vascular disease, a commonly associated complication of diabetes mellitus. It is easy to understand, then, why diabetics are at particular risk for heart attacks and strokes.

Type I, often known as "juvenile diabetes," is more common, seen in two thousand out of one hundred thousand people in the United States, and is the type that usually

requires insulin injections. Type II, which does not require insulin injections, is seen in about two per one thousand people in the United States. Type II usually is not diagnosed until adulthood, and is often associated with obesity.

Both types tend to run in families. In fact, some kind of family history can be found for 25 percent of diabetics. If you find diabetes on your family tree, try to learn if it is Type I (insulin-dependent) or Type II. If a family member is being treated for diabetes, other family members should have their blood-sugar levels checked regularly.

SMOKING: MORE GENETIC THAN YOU THINK?

For years we have heard about the "addictive" personality and how there is a genetic link in many cases, including alcoholism, drug abuse, and a variety of psychiatric problems.

But now researchers are adding another behavior to this list of addictive personalities—cigarette smoking. This is news because it puts smokers in a new category: prisoners of their own genetic cells. In the past, smokers have been viewed simply as people with a bad habit. Since the Surgeon General's report on the health dangers of smoking came out in 1966, the number of smokers has steadily decreased. And as smoking has become less "politically correct" in public and social situations, it is believed that casual smoking has declined substantially.

What we are left with are the hard-core smokers, those who are addicted to nicotine and find it nearly impossible to quit. Scientists studying possible genetic links in smoking behavior are now focusing on this group.

Researchers for the National Institutes of Mental Health have come up with some fascinating findings: People who smoke are more than twice as likely to suffer from a major depression at some point in their lives.

Another group of scientists (at the Ford Health Sciences Center in Detroit) interviewed one thousand young-adult smokers and came up with a reverse proposition: that people with a history of depression are twice as likely to become hooked on nicotine than smokers without a history of depression.

So we are left with the classic chicken-or-the-egg question: Which comes first, the depression or the smoking? What many scientists are now saying is surprising. Both come at the same time, possibly the result of the same genetic markers!

There is a logical theory that nicotine has a euphoric effect that may temporarily lift a person from depression. But it is more likely, scientists now say, that the craving for nicotine may be the body's way of compensating for genes that may be missing in people with chronic depression. Could there be the same genetic predisposition for both disorders? This could explain why stop-smoking clinics have only a 30 percent success rate after one year. If hereditary factors play a part in nicotine addiction, the habit is all that much harder to kick.

This theory is hard to take for many veteran smokers. They have never been labeled as "sick" before, the way we label other problems of addiction. But many researchers now firmly believe that smoking, depression, and substance abuse are inextricably linked, possibly by the same gene or set of genes.

But your tendency to get lung cancer from smoking might not be as genetic as you think. A study published in August 1994 looked at 681 pairs of male twins in which one brother smoked and died of lung cancer. It found that most of their twin brothers, who also smoked, did not die of the disease.

Scientists at the National Cancer Institute, which did the study, say if a smoker thinks it is okay to continue the habit because his smoking parents did not get lung cancer, he could be making a fatal assumption. The study, while controversial, points out the necessity of including lifestyle information while compiling your medical family tree.

I'll have more on the genetics of addictive behavior in the next chapter.

Each relative or ancestor with heart disease has a different set of circumstances. For each known case of heart disease on your family tree, answer as many of these questions as possible:

DID RELATIVE/ANCESTOR . . .	RISK OF GENETIC LINK EVEN GREATER IF . . .
• have a heart attack?	• under the age of sixty
• take medication for angina (chest pain caused by partially blocked arteries). At what age was he or she diagnosed with angina?	• medication necessary under the age of sixty
• take medication for hypertension (high blood pressure)? Hypertension causes damage to artery walls, and thus allows fatty deposits to collect. It is believed to be connected to the metabolism of sodium.	• there appears to be an inherited predisposition to hypertension. People with high blood pressure have at least a three times greater risk of heart disease.
• have atherosclerosis (hardening of the arteries)? At what age?	• diagnosed under the age of sixty. There is a strong inherited predisposition to factors causing atherosclerosis, but there are also environmental causes (such as smoking or a fatty diet).
• have rheumatic fever as a child?	• there's no history of rheumatic fever (which can cause heart irregularities).
• have a stroke? At what age?	• happened under the age of sixty. A stroke happens because the cardiovascular system is clogged. If it occurs earlier in life, the cause might involve genetic factors.
• have high blood cholesterol or a rare genetic defect called "hypercholesterolemia"?	• diagnosed with high blood cholesterol at any age. The tendency to have high cholesterol can be inherited. "Hypercholesterolemia" definitely runs in families.
• have a history of diabetes mellitus (insulin-dependent)	• insulin-dependent at any age. 25 percent of insulin-dependent diabetics have a family history of diabetes, and 75 percent of diabetics die from vascular disease.
• have coronary bypass surgery? At what age?	• coronary bypass occurs under the age of sixty. Bypass surgery means there was severe blockage of the arteries. Factors leading to blockage could be genetic.
• have history of low plasminogen activator levels? This is a blood-clot dissolver.	• low plasminogen activator levels are diagnosed at any age. A plasminogen activator shortage runs in families.
• have an enlarged heart?	• enlarged heart is diagnosed at any age. Recent studies shows this potentially dangerous condition probably has genetic links.

LIFESTYLE INFORMATION

After completing as many of the above questions as possible, you are ready to add environmental and lifestyle information to your medical family tree. Some of the questions below may be similar to those covered earlier concerning cancer and other illnesses, but if they are specifically relevant to heart disease, I will repeat them here.

Answer these questions about each relative or ancestor with heart disease.

1. Was relative a smoker? How long?

    WHY IMPORTANT: Smoking has for years been linked to heart disease. Relative's heart problems could be caused by his or her lifestyle, not necessarily genetics.

    Was relative an ex-smoker (must have stopped for at least a year)?

    WHY IMPORTANT: The more years your relative was an ex-smoker, the less likely that his or her heart disease was caused by lifestyle, although it is still possible.

2. What do you know about relative's weight? By each name on your medical family tree, write "thin," "average," "overweight," or "obese.

    WHY IMPORTANT: People who are obese have a greater tendency toward high cholesterol. However, if your relatives are of normal weight and have a history of high cholesterol, the cause is more likely to be genetic.

3. What do you know about relative's drinking habits? For each relative, indicate "nondrinker," "moderate drinker," or "heavy drinker." ("Heavy drinker" would be daily drinking, more than three ounces of alcohol per drink.)

    WHY IMPORTANT: Heavy drinking can cause high blood pressure and increased heart rate, which can eventually damage the heart. Your relative's heart disease could be caused by lifestyle, or a combination of genetics and lifestyle.

4. Illicit drug use? Which drug(s)?

    WHY IMPORTANT: If relative used cocaine, marijuana, anabolic steroids, or other illicit drugs, that lifestyle choice alone could cause heart damage. This is difficult to trace but worth noting on your medical family tree if you have the information.

5. How much did relative exercise?

    Write "never exercised," "sometimes exercised," or "regular exercise" by each relative's name on your medical family tree. (Regular exercise means at least three times a week, at least twenty minutes a session.)

    WHY IMPORTANT: If relative took good care of self by regular exercise, heart disease could be genetic, and *not* caused by lifestyle factors.

How Do I Analyze the Heart Disease on My Medical Family Tree?

Because heart disease is a unique blend of genetic and environmental (or lifestyle) factors, a good analysis of the heart problems on your tree requires deft juggling.

If there is no smoking, heavy drinking, or obesity in the family, you can guess that any family heart disease might be genetic.

On the contrary, if there is smoking, drinking, obesity and *no* heart disease, you might be at lower risk than most people.

In the long haul, it really doesn't matter if a family tendency toward heart disease is more environmental than genetic, or the other way around. If you see any kind of pattern, it is a warning, and it means you should consult with your doctor about lifestyle changes.

If you can determine a probable family link, use the knowledge as a weapon against poor health. A genetic risk is all the more reason to be careful and have frequent, aggressive check-ups with a cardiologist. And you may want to inform other family members to do the same. *It is your future. Only you can try to change your genetic destiny or family legacy.*

HEART DISEASE: SEPARATING NATURE FROM NURTURE

S o you've done your medical family tree, and gasp, you see heart attacks all over the place. "I'm doomed," you might think. Why even bother with a diet of veggie burgers and bean sprouts?

A study by the National Heart, Lung and Blood Institute has a confusing answer to that dilemma. It has been tracking 514 white male twin pairs who are veterans from World War II and the Korean War. Some are identical twins (who have exactly the same genes) and some are fraternal twins (who, on the average, have 50 percent of the same genes, the same percentage as any siblings).

If heredity really mattered in heart disease, wouldn't the heart problems be worse among the identical twins? If one identical twin has heart problems, doesn't the other one have a greater chance of getting it than in the case of fraternal twins, who come from two separate eggs?

Researchers found there was little difference between rates of heart disease in the two different types of twins. This, of course, underscores the important role of environment, because all of these sets of twins grew up in the same households, presumably with similar lifestyles and eating habits.

But even the researchers admit the study is flawed. It only followed twins who were healthy enough to be in the military in the first place, and it began after the twins turned forty, eliminating any twins who may have had heart disease prior to that age.

But researchers did learn one interesting fact: There was a higher rate of heart disease among twins than among other members of their family. So scientists looking at heart disease still haven't figured out how much is genetic, how much is lifestyle, and how these two interact to make a person sick.

INHERITED HEART DISEASE: TWO PERSONAL STORIES

Harold

It was a warm summer day and Harold Board was mowing the lawn at his home in Greenville, Indiana. He had just passed his forty-eighth birthday. Harold was a busy man, a principal at an elementary school. He had a healthy past and an energetic life with his wife and two children. But his grass-cutting was interrupted by an inexplicable burning sensation across his chest. "No pain," said Harold, "just a weird burning."

Harold considered himself to be an educated man on such matters. After all, first aid is part of any teacher's training. So he dutifully went to his family doctor.

"Let's do an EKG," said the doctor. Again, a seemingly proper response. But the doctor told him it wasn't a heart attack at all. The electrocardiogram and follow-up exam showed nothing more than inflamed bronchial tubes. Harold was sent home.

This is the point where one's personal knowledge can alter one's fate. If Harold had studied his medical family tree at the first hint of trouble, he might have made different choices in his life.

Instead, he didn't think much about it and continued his smoking habit. He was relieved he could continue his work as principal at the V. O. Isom Elementary School in Greenville. "Kids have a tough way to go these days," he told me. "They need more guidance and more caring because they often don't have what they need at home."

Two years after the "bronchial" incident, Harold was working in his home workshop. It was Easter Sunday and he wanted to make good use of every second at home. Again, he felt that burning feeling. This time it was so severe Harold lay down on his couch. He could feel his heart beating as fast as a locomotive. As Harold rested, he thought of his father, who dropped dead of a heart attack while baling hay at the family farm when he was just fifty-two years old. Harold was fifty and scared.

The doctor ordered an EKG and a treadmill test and, surprisingly, Harold passed both with honors. "That is 90 percent proof," the doctor told him, "that your heart is fine." Harold went home again. But he couldn't shake the memory of his father. He put together an informal medical family tree, concentrating on heart disease patterns.

Harold was surprised at what he saw. He knew that every family had its share of heart attacks and cardiovascular problems. But on his family tree he saw a pattern of heart problems at relatively young ages. His mother was still alive at eight-two, after heart bypass surgery at seventy-six. But when he asked his mother when her heart problems started she answered, "In my late fifties." Apparently she was diagnosed with an enlarged heart and high blood pressure, was given medication, and proved to be an ideal patient.

Harold knew that his grandfather Frank, on his mother's side, died of a stroke at seventy-two. But it wasn't until he put together his medical family tree that he learned Frank had had three brothers who had died of heart attacks at early ages. One of them, Tom, died in his early thirties.

Harold's grandmother on his mother's side, Clara, died of cancer in her seventies. But while probing for more information, Harold learned

Clara had a brother, Raymond, who died at forty-seven of a heart attack.

Harold was not yet fifty but began to really worry about his future health. He seemed fine, but did have that smoking habit. He took the family tree to Dr. Buzz Hickman, a cardiologist at the University of Indiana Medical Center.

"Dr. Hickman said he had a gut feeling that I was in danger," says Harold, "but it was the family history that convinced the doctor to look further."

"He was right. He did a heart catheter test and found what the other doctors hadn't been able to find: significant blockage in my arteries. He said I would probably have to have surgery sometime in the next five years."

Harold went home in a state of shock, but was relieved he wasn't just imagining all those symptoms. He settled back into his work at his school and thought he had a few years before his health would be in real danger. Even now, he underestimated the strong messages in his medical family tree.

One night, about a year later, Harold says he began to have a very "nervous" feeling. "I was tired enough to sleep, but for some strange reason I couldn't sit down. I took a sleeping pill and a Valium, but I still felt like I was ready to explode. I began to sweat, my stomach felt awful, I took some antacids. I would get this feeling of tightness throughout my body for a while, then it would just float away."

Astonishingly, Harold drove himself to the doctor, who immediately put him in a hospital. "You've had a heart attack," the doctor told him, "and you're going into surgery."

That day Harold had five bypasses on his heart, five blocked arteries given new life, reconstructed and sewn onto unobstructed parts of his heart for a cleaner blood flow. But that's not the end of the story.

Harold passed his fifty-second birthday and breathed a sigh of relief that his doctor's aggressive action spared him from his father's fate. He was so confident of his recovery, he continued his smoking habit and decided not to look reality in the eye. "Not that I didn't try to stop," he tells me. "I did hypnosis, clinics, nicotine gum, the whole bit."

But in the back of his mind, he wondered if he could really live as long as his mother, or if he would share his father's legacy of dying young.

One morning, about six and a half years after

FAMILIES WITH BIG HEARTS ARE MORE THAN JUST GENEROUS

*T*here is a mysterious and sometimes deadly disease of the heart called "cardiomyopathy," commonly known as an enlarged heart. When the chambers of the heart enlarge, blood is not pumped efficiently. In some cases, a virus or alcohol abuse can cause the lower chambers to swell, but often there is no known cause.

Recently, a team of researchers at the Mayo Clinic discovered a familial link with the disorder. Nature or lifestyle? Researchers want to find out and are looking for a guilty gene. Whatever they discover, the new evidence should encourage people with a family history of cardiomyopathy to get a special test called an "echocardiogram."

While many people don't know they have this disorder until it's too late, some typical symptoms are: extreme weakness and shortness of breath. This is another important reason to know your family health history.

Harold Board Looks at His Family's Heart Disease

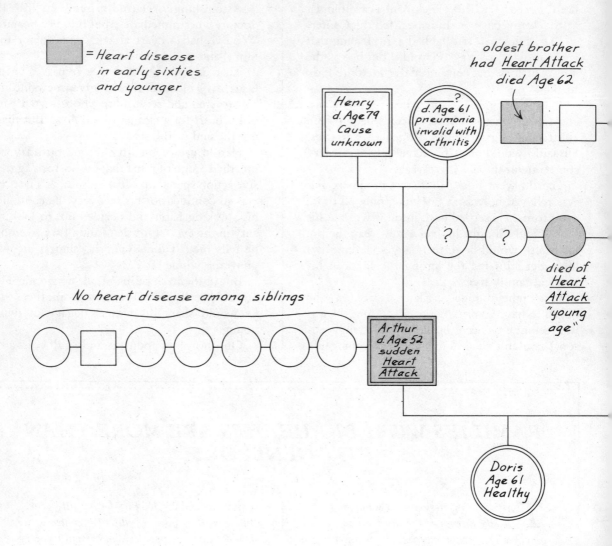

= Heart disease in early sixties and younger

oldest brother had *Heart Attack* died Age 62

Henry d. Age 79 Cause unknown

? d. Age 61 pneumonia invalid with arthritis

? ?

died of *Heart Attack* "young age"

No heart disease among siblings

Arthur d. Age 52 sudden *Heart Attack*

Doris Age 61 Healthy

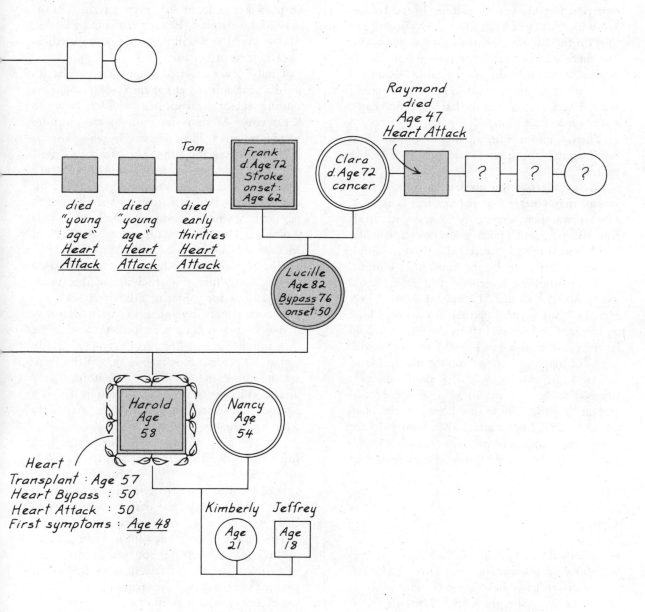

his surgery, Harold awoke and knew something was wrong. Soon he was in the hospital for another bypass operation. But this time his recovery was slow. "I couldn't breathe," he says. "I was constantly gasping, coughing. I hadn't thought about dying, but I knew things weren't going well." Harold put out his last cigarette.

In fact, at a relatively young age, Harold was experiencing slow and painful heart failure, known as ischemic heart disease. His doctor put him on the list for a heart transplant program, but there was no guarantee they would find a heart. "It was torture," says Harold. "I waited three months for a heart, every day getting weaker and weaker. For the last forty-two days, I was on a heart pump."

Then, without warning, his doctor burst into his hospital room and said, "We've got a match."

Today Harold is back on the job, with a young man's heart that is pumping with ease. He knows there are no promises with heart transplants, but he's taken a new direction in life.

"I look at life a lot differently," says Harold. "Every day my feet hit the floor, it's a bonus."

Was it smoking or genetics that gave Harold his brush with death? "I'll never be sure," says Harold, "but I wish I had taken a detailed look at the family history earlier. Maybe it would have been the incentive I needed to stop smoking. But thank goodness I did the medical family tree, because it was the single greatest motivation to seek expert help. The cardiologist at Indiana University kept me one step ahead of a fatal heart attack. My family doctor didn't even ask about my family history in detail. If I had stuck with him, I'd probably be dead."

Cindy

Now let's take a look at one lucky (and smart) woman who got a warning at a young enough age to control her heart's health. Her name is Cindy Leffew. She grew up in Danville, Kentucky, in a family full of heavy smokers. At a young age, she, too, started the habit. And like many young people, she wasn't especially careful about what she ate.

Six years ago, Cindy's mother Beverly was trying to climb a flight of stairs in her home. Beverly was only forty-three years old, so she didn't suspect anything serious when she became breathless. But when it happened a second time, Beverly had to lie down. Cindy insisted on calling an ambulance. Paramedics suspected trouble, and they were right. On the way to the hospital, Beverly had a heart attack. She survived and will probably be on medication the rest of her life.

Cindy never worried about her own health until a year ago, when, at thirty-one, she felt a burning sensation from her shoulders down to her wrists. At first she thought the episodes were infrequent, but then they began to last for several minutes at a time. She had been suffering from pneumonia and assumed it was a symptom of that. But she pieced together a bit of her family health history and showed it to her doctor, who immediately sent her to a cardiologist, Dr. Mark Turrentine, at Wishard Memorial Hospital in Indianapolis.

The first few tests showed little, but based on her family history (which included an uncle who died at forty-five of a heart attack), her new doctor was very aggressive in his diagnostic work-up and did a heart catheter test. What they found was startling. At thirty-one, Cindy had an 80 percent blockage in one of the main arteries supplying the heart. She immediately underwent bypass surgery. Although it was a painful experience, she views it as a friendly warning signal.

Today Cindy is doing well. She has stopped smoking, eats a low-fat diet, and has her kids on the same regime. "When Mom had a heart attack, I learned how to cook low-cholesterol foods for her, so it was easy to adapt—especially when you're looking death in the face."

Her family history has kept her anxious in a positive way. When her son was complaining of a pain in his chest a few months ago, some people thought it was "psychological," as if he were mimicking his mother's experience.

But Cindy took it seriously and had him tested. Doctors discovered an irregular heartbeat (commonly called a "heart murmur"), which seems to run in her family at early ages. Heart murmurs are usually not serious, but now the whole family is being closely watched. But Cindy is still very concerned. Some family members are experiencing denial,

and they continue to smoke and have poor eating habits.

"Not me," says Cindy, who, thanks to her medical family tree, took action and possibly was spared a heart attack. "Never again will I take life for granted."

STEP SIX
Find the Right Specialist

No one can complete the perfect family tree—information will always be missing or hard to get. But even partial information can be lifesaving in the right hands. If you see any patterns or "red flags," make an appointment with a medical geneticist at the nearest university medical center (even if you have to drive a few hours to get there).

You should also make an appointment with a specialist who treats the disease most prevalent on your medical family tree. A consultation will benefit not only you but everyone in your family. If these specially trained doctors

see a potentially dangerous pattern, they may want to order the appropriate tests on a regular basis.

Many family doctors and physicians at community hospitals are trained in genetics, but I encourage your first consultation to be with a doctor at a major medical center. Because these centers are usually teaching and research hospitals, they are more up-to-date with the latest findings in this exciting, cutting-edge field. Just three years ago, one of my sisters encountered a family doctor who was still unaware that ovarian cancer could be hereditary!

THERE ARE GOOD GENES TOO!

*T*he genetic research explosion is not just uncovering dangerous genes. There is a little gem called "p53" that actually suppresses the development of cancer. The p53 gene (named for its location in the chromosomal structure) is the enforcer gene, keeping the body's cells in their proper place.

The p53 gene creates a protein in the cell that can sense the first signs of damage to the chromosomes. Scientists repeatedly have found that the gene is mutated or absent when certain cancers are present. This could lead to better and earlier cancer diagnosis. If p53 is absent in certain tissue samples, it could mean that cancer is on its way.

Even more intriguing is a report in the July 1994 issue of the medical journal Cell

that says cancer patients with thriving p53 genes respond best to radiation and chemotherapy. If doctors could determine which patients carry this miniature arsenal, they could better predict who will do well with conventional treatment. If a patient does not have an intact p53, more aggressive treatments could be tried sooner, sparing the patient months, even years, of difficult side effects.

Think of the possibilities! If scientists learn to repair the mutated p53 gene or replace an absent p53 gene, could the damaged, cancer-stricken tissue reverse itself and heal? Doctors at the M. D. Anderson Cancer Center in Houston are now experimenting with this revolutionary treatment on lung cancer patients. Watch for the results.

Cindy Leffew's Medical Family Tree

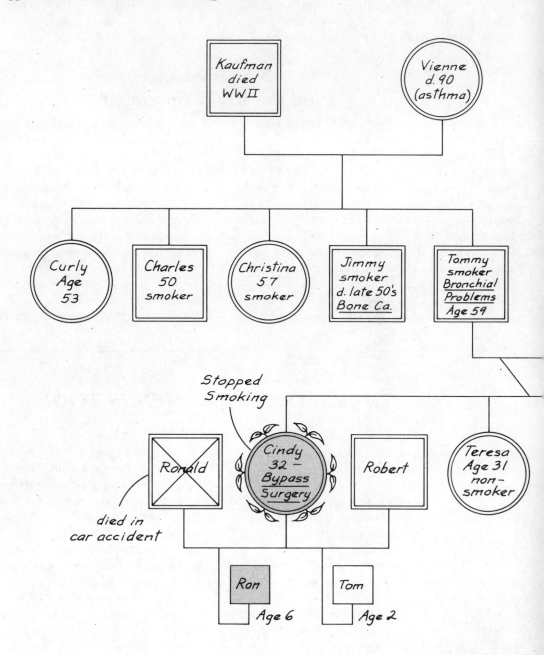

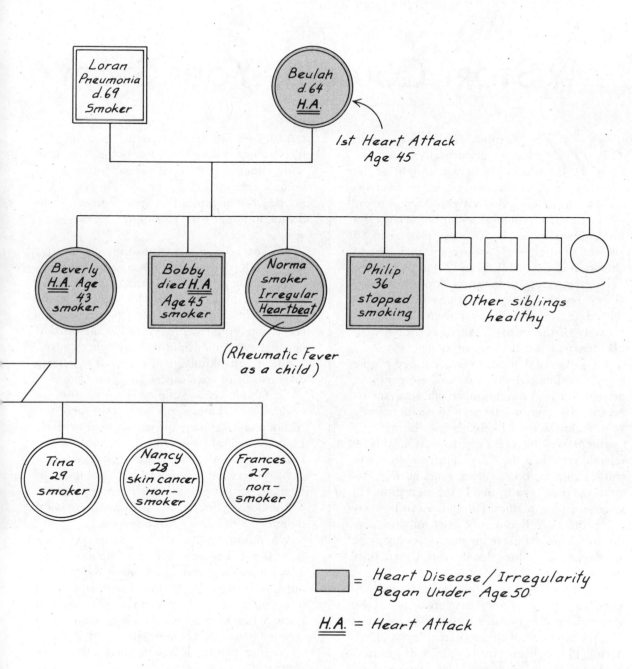

Cindy was careful to find out who was a smoker and who wasn't. Her aunt Norma has heart problems, but she had rheumatic fever as a child, which could be the cause. The more information on a medical family tree, the easier it is for a doctor to analyze it.

MY STORY COULD BE YOUR STORY

My family's story may soon change dramatically with the discovery of what might be the sinister gene that has caused our colon, ovarian, and uterine cancers. A study published last year by doctors from Johns Hopkins University and the University of Helsinki says that 65 to 80 percent of the people who carry an inherited alteration in the "MSH2" or "MHL1" gene are likely to develop colon cancer. Most of the rest who carry this dangerous gene will develop a related cancer, usually ovarian or uterine but possibly of the stomach, small intentines, gall bladder, pancrea, urethra, or kidney.

It is believed that.one in two hundred people carry the inherited alteration of these genes. A genetic test is in development, and soon members of my family will have to decide if they want to know their likely genetic destiny.

But it will be years before we know how reliable tests like these are, since scientists are still looking for other culprit genes in this devastating family syndrome. In the meantime, researching your medical family tree can be your best protection. Becauses of my family history, my son Zack will have his first colonoscopy at age twenty-five, three decades earlier than most people.

For people like Zack, full of energy and potential, a personal medical map can help lead the way to a healthy journey through life long before we uncover all the mysteries of the DNA strand. If you learn you have a predisposition for hypertension, you may have the incentive you need to throw away the salt shaker. If your family has a history of high cholesterol, you are likely to take warnings about diet more seriously. A young couple with a checkered med-ical background can get genetic counseling before having children of their own. A woman with a family pattern of breast cancer might become religious about breast self-exams and not skip her mammogram appointments. Your doctor and your own passion for life can guide you.

My sister Susan and I are still free of cancer. My sister Kathy, who four years ago faced late-stage ovarian cancer, is still successfully battling the disease. My cousin Barb has outlived all the normal odds for a diagnosis of pancreatic cancer, and recently was overjoyed at the birth of her first two grandchildren. My other cousin, Joanie, is, thankfully, still cancer-free, after a diagnosis of ovarian cancer two years ago.

Susan and I have adopted the little girls we couldn't bear biologically after our surgeries. Although I have many questions about my little Emma's medical family tree, I am comforted to know she doesn't share any of my genes!

My sisters and I (and our five biological children) are still at risk for other cancers, but we will undergo periodic and painstaking medical monitoring for the rest of our lives.

No mortal individual can intervene when one's fate is determined. But where destiny allows some maneuvering, it is up to you to maximize your chances for a long life. Think about it. If you were standing on a railroad track and knew a freight train was coming, would you stay on the track or try to jump off in time?

For my family, it has become an issue of control. Researching our family's medical history let us know the train was coming. At least we know we are doing all we can.

A medical family tree can give you power over your future.

IV

Your Behavioral Family Tree

The twentieth century was the century of Freud;
the twenty-first century is going to be the century
of genes as far as behavior is concerned.

DR. DAVID E. COMINGS
CITY OF HOPE NATIONAL MEDICAL CENTER,
DUARTE, CALIFORNIA

DISCOVERING YOUR GENOGRAM

*S*everal months ago a friend of mine I'll call Samuel confessed to me that he was struggling with feelings of unexplained anger and intolerance toward others in his life.

On the surface, this was easy to understand. Eight years ago Samuel went into treatment for alcoholism, an addiction that had cost him his job. But with his extraordinary intelligence and consummate perfectionism, he tackled his addiction with vigor. He is still sober today, has a terrific wife, and two great kids. He's also back at work as a producer in Hollywood, a town known for its forgiving attitudes only when it comes to doing time at rehabilitation centers.

So why the anger? After several years of therapy, Samuel concluded that he had experienced a pretty decent childhood. There had been no overt trauma, no physical or sexual abuse, his parents were affluent and had given him pretty much what he wanted. He wondered if his alcoholism stemmed from feelings of inadequacy, despite his career success. Because he was not able to find the source of his anger, he stopped seeing a therapist and philosophized that he might never know the answers.

I suggested to Samuel that he try to construct a genogram, a sort of behavioral family tree that traces patterns of emotions, communications, and coping methods over three or more generations. Unlike a medical family tree, a genogram does not rely on official records or medical documents. Instead, it uses subjective reports of communication patterns, major life events, and illnesses to help people visualize their lives in the context of their families.

A genogram can shed light on the way family members have related to one another through the years. Once you discover patterns that have not worked well, you can act to change them. Even more exciting, you can learn how to use your family's strengths.

Genograms have been around for about fifteen years, but have been used mostly by professional therapists. The genogram format was conceived by family therapist Murray Bowen, a legendary figure in the field.

Bowen concluded (partly from experiments on his own family) that mental health evolves when a person makes decisions outside of and apart from certain family pressures.

I contacted Larry Mauksch, a family psychotherapist and behavioral scientist at the University of Washington Department of Family Medicine in Seattle. Mauksch has been writing and teaching about genograms to help people better understand their behavior. He generously agreed to work with Samuel and me to come up with a genogram model that Samuel could use to help him manage and accept his life more, by looking at family patterns. "I will not be your therapist," Mauksch told Samuel. "You will be the one doing the work."

What evolved from our work together is what I call a consumer model of a genogram: an application you can use to help unlock the subtle and sometimes mysterious influence your family had—and still has—on you. You may be surprised at how much your extended family helps to mold your emotions and reactions.

But the genogram model comes with a warning: "If in the process you feel uncontrolled pain or anxiety, it would be wise to consult a therapist, who can help you understand the genogram," Mauksch advises. "It is possible that you will make a discovery or come to a conclusion that will startle you and be painful. It is a good idea to be prepared. And a therapist can be a neutral, nonjudgmental friend who can help you understand your family dynamics."

HOW DO I BEGIN?

*I*t is easy to begin a genogram. Copy the basics of a block graph family tree onto a separate, large paper (see pages 26–27 and 149). Start with three generations. You and your siblings, your parents, and your grandparents. Add a fourth generation if you have children. Use squares for males, circles for females. Include nonrelatives who've played important roles in your family. Let's see how Samuel's genogram unfolded before you begin your own.

Include when possible:
Names
Ages (dates of birth)
Causes of death

Samuel's beginning genogram can be seen on page 108–9.

Then our expert, Mauksch, asked Samuel to describe core issues of his life. "Is there something you would like to better understand about yourself—an area of pain—something you question about yourself?"

Mauksch's query was interesting to me because we, of course, all have issues of pain in our lives. But usually they sit on our shoulders with some vague and ever-changing distribution of weight, escaping our full view. To be asked to clearly define each area of pain is indeed a difficult, possibly hurtful chore. I was anxious to hear Samuel's answer.

"I would really like to work on accepting myself the way that I am," Samuel told us. "And I would like to accept others better, not get so angry inside. I would like to learn to manage my anger and be more tolerant of life as it changes." Mauksch summarized Samuel's core issues into three categories: "Anger," "Tolerance," and "Lack of self-acceptance."

As an observer of this process, this raised my curiosity further. I wondered what my core issues would be. Certainly, each of us is an exceptional human being, but we must each explore how our uniqueness merges with others. To make a genogram work, we must use it to come to terms with our behavior as it relates to those closest to us and as it spins out into the greater world.

For that reason, I will refer to Samuel's key issues as "painpoints." His goal will not be to judge his behavior or magically erase the pain in his life. Instead, the genogram should help him decode the mystery of his behavior, so he can learn to better anticipate and control his emotional responses.

Now that Samuel's painpoints have been clearly identified, it's time to get back to work on the genogram. For that, we go back to our expert, Larry Mauksch. "Make a list," he told Samuel, "of any major life events that have affected your family. These would be milestones or moments that may have rippled down to others. Births, deaths, marriages, separations, the end of long-term relationships, moves, job

YOUR OWN GENOGRAM WORKBOOK BEGINS ON PAGE 147

changes, and so on. If anything comes to mind, trust your instincts," Mauksch insisted, "don't analyze it. After you make your list, mark the events at the appropriate places on your genogram, using whatever abbreviations you want."

As we see on pages 110–11 Samuel's genogram began to take a new form.

Mauksch continued his instructions: "Take the genogram and add major diseases and note what impact they had on the family. Then, note major mental illness or emotional issues. Remember, you are not a mental health professional, just write down what comes from within you, even if it's a hunch." Samuel's genogram began to look more intricate: (See pages 112–13)

As he began to ponder Mauksch's latest suggestions, I looked closely over Samuel's shoulder at the genogram he was creating. I noticed he had not marked down any siblings for his grandparents. "Anything you might have left out?" I asked, pointing to the upper tier of relatives.

"Nothing significant, really," Samuel answered. "My grandma Dora did have some siblings but they all died before I was born, so I can't really see how they could have affected us."

"How did they die?" I asked.

"In concentration camps in Poland during World War II."

"And you're not sure if this is significant?" I asked.

"Is it?" Samuel answered, his eyes filling with astonishment and understanding.

"Samuel," I said, "write it down so we can look at the whole picture."

Later Larry Mauksch would tell us, "Your discovery of the effect of the Holocaust on Samuel's family is important, and it came by noticing the conspicuous absence of information."

Samuel's addition to his genogram put a whole new tilt to his family dynamics. (Pages 114–15)

Then Mauksch asked Samuel to go back to what I defined as his painpoints: anger, tolerance, and self-acceptance. "Think of each person and the tree in the context of these issues," he told Samuel. "Does anything ring a bell? Did anyone have a problem with anger, at themselves, at you, or someone else in the family or outside the family? And what about basic tolerance of others in the family or outside the home? What about acceptance? Did anyone have a problem accepting you or others? Do they still? Make a mark or a note when something clicks."

Samuel realized the easy part was over. This assignment required calm and serious thought. Over a period of days, he began to write down pieces of his family life that seemed to relate somehow to his painpoints. This is where a genogram must stay open-ended. Don't confine yourself to a one-page format. Even when you think you are done, more information and insight almost always emerge.

Here are some of the key points in Samuel's analysis of his painpoints and his family:

ON ANGER: "Mother and I used to fight often. She has an angry, embittered side and [since I was] the oldest, I seemed to take the brunt of it." My father and I would fight less, but the fights were more intense than they were with my mother.

"Of all my grandparents, I only really knew Grandma Dora, my mother's mom. She is really an awful person, angry and mean-spirited toward my mother, but usually very nice to me.

"My cousins, Dorothy's kids, seem to have a lot of anger toward me. I think they resent the fact my mother refused to take Grandma Dora in when she became old and ill. This may be just an extension of the resentment and anger between my mother and her siblings on this issue. My mother does help Grandma out financially, but I think that's part of the resentment, that we are more affluent than they are. My cousin Susan on my father's side also seems envious and never seems to be friendly or have a nice word. My reaction is to ignore her."

ON TOLERANCE: "There seems to be a guilt system in the family that makes tolerance difficult. My father and his brothers are always working so hard for their business that they get resentful when someone takes time off.

"Also, everyone is expected to be at family gatherings and rituals . . . you're made to feel guilty if you aren't. If you act the way the rest of the family acts about these things, you're tolerated. If you say, 'No, I want to spend time with my wife and children this weekend,' it simply isn't tolerated. Also, incompetence on the job is not tolerated. When I was fired from my job, my parents were embarrassed, as if their own pride was severely damaged. And for a while, they were in complete denial over my alcoholism. They simply couldn't tolerate such poor behavior from their son. In the end they began to understand."

ON SELF-ACCEPTANCE: "I was only accepted by my parents when I played by their rules.

"My mother was never accepting of my dad's obsession with the business, and she felt neglected. This, along with her conflicts with her own mother, makes her feel guilty, and she doesn't like herself for these feelings. I think my mother feels guilty about putting my brother Peter in an institution.

"My cousins Cynthia and Jane (Dorothy's kids on my mom's side) seem to have a chip on their shoulder. They seem envious of my career success and the greater affluence of my family. I think it reflects their parents' attitude toward my parents.

"I have trouble accepting myself in relation to my wife Jennifer. She thinks I am too bound by family obligations, that I don't think for myself enough. Jennifer has made me stronger and has helped me to separate in a healthy way from my family, but I worry I'll stray too far and feel guilty about that. I always feel inadequate in relation to my children, who much prefer their mother."

For the next step, Mauksch recommended that Samuel describe the relationships that existed between key people on his tree. He noted the general categories that Samuel could use:

1. **CLOSE:** Intimate, mutually supportive relationship that doesn't sacrifice appreciation of individual differences.
2. **FUSED (OVERLY CLOSE):** Inhibiting identification and expression of individual thoughts and feelings (some people might describe this as "smothering").
3. **DISTANT:** Not much contact or conflict.
4. **CONFLICTUAL:** Not intimate; argumentative.
5. **FUSED AND CONFLICTUAL:** Neither one knowing how to function individually or to respect the needs of the other to do so.
6. **CUT OFF:** Not talking or not tolerating.

IN YOUR HEART'S MEMORY

*W*hen making a genogram, relax and go *with your instincts. If a family incident seemed small, but it somehow sticks in your mind, write it down. If you suspect that your family was somehow impacted by an event in your life, but you aren't really sure, make a note of it.*

"Don't analyze anything, just trust your gut and listen to yourself," says Larry Mauksch. "You have certain senses, images. I call it 'Strong-in-Your-Heart's-Memory.' You don't have to rationalize or document it, just write it down."

Mauksch stresses that a genogram can be an emotional experience. Throughout the process, if you feel a certain emotion, make a note of it. If your painpoint is your uncontrolled anger, for example, it is important to note at which point in the process you feel anger. "Don't try to explain it, just note the feeling," he tells us.

Mauksch suggested Samuel not worry about exact definitions of each category and choose the description that seemed to fit best.

Because relationships change over the years, Mauksch also suggested Samuel make judgments based on when relationships were strongest and note what turn of events changed the relationship. "Don't necessarily look at the state of the relationship right now," said Mauksch, "but rather how it lives in your history. For example, your parents may get along well now, but maybe they didn't when you were growing up. In other words, describe those relationships that were strongest in your heart's memory."

For this, Samuel would need a certain genogram "language," which we have adapted partly from symbols standardized by the Task Force of the North America Primary Care Research Group chaired by Monica McGoldrick, M.S.W., a pioneer in genogram development.

Close ———————————————

Fused. ═══════════════════════

Conflictual ∧∨∧∨∧∨∧∨∧∨

Fused and conflictual ⩓⩓⩓⩓⩓⩓

Distant – – – – – – – – – – – – –

Cut off —⊣ ⊢—⊣ ⊢—⊣ ⊢—

Making the Genogram Readable

To make Samuel's genogram easier to put together, he first noted his relationships with others on the chart, then on separate charts he noted his perception of his mother's and father's relationships. In a really complicated genogram you could continue the process among all your relatives, if their relationships seemed to impact on you significantly. The next series of illustrations is the result of Samuel's thoughtful work:

DEPRESSION

*D*epression is defined in the American Medical Association's Encyclopedia of Medicine *as "feelings of sadness, hopelessness, and a general loss of interest in life, combined with a sense of reduced emotional wellbeing."*

Most of us have experienced those feelings to some extent, usually after a difficult or tragic event. But when these feelings deepen for no apparent cause, and won't go away, it could be a more serious psychiatric illness. This kind of clinical depression is linked to low levels of the brain neurotransmitter, serotonin. The newer antidepressant drugs, such as the popular Prozac, have been successful in treating some depression by increasing serotonin levels. This is a different approach to the treatment of depression, which in years past has been treated by strong sedatives, making the patient lethargic and drowsy. In a handful of well-publicized cases, some people have claimed they experienced extreme behavioral reaction to drugs like Prozac. But by and large it is being used by hundreds of thousands of psychiatric patients who swear by its effectiveness.

More and more evidence is piling up to support the theory that the tendency toward depression is genetic. A recent study at the National Institute of Mental Health shows that people biologically related to someone with clinical depression are twice as likely to experience depression than are the relatives of nondepressed people. This study was done on people who were adopted and raised outside of their biological family environments.

Depression clearly runs in families. It is a good reason to log your family behavioral history and get your situation analyzed by a psychiatrist or family therapist. There are effective ways to intervene, and a clear picture of your family can help guide your treatment.

Samuel's Beginning Genogram

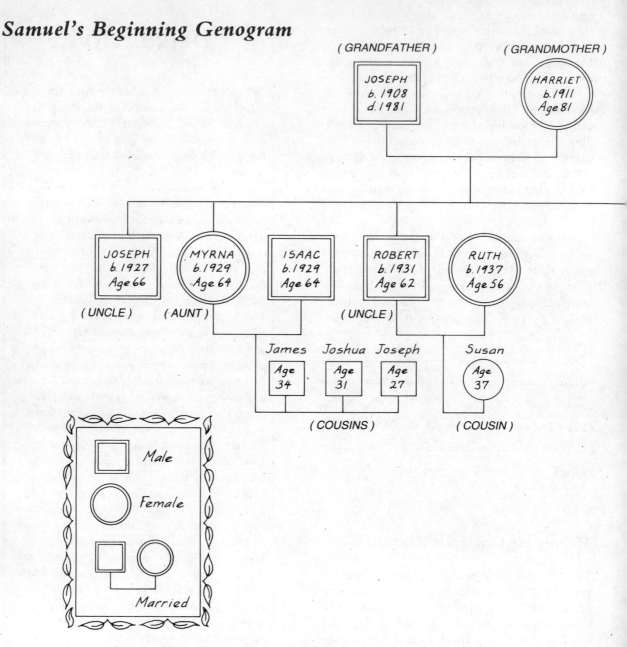

Names and some identical facts have been changed
to protect the family's privacy.

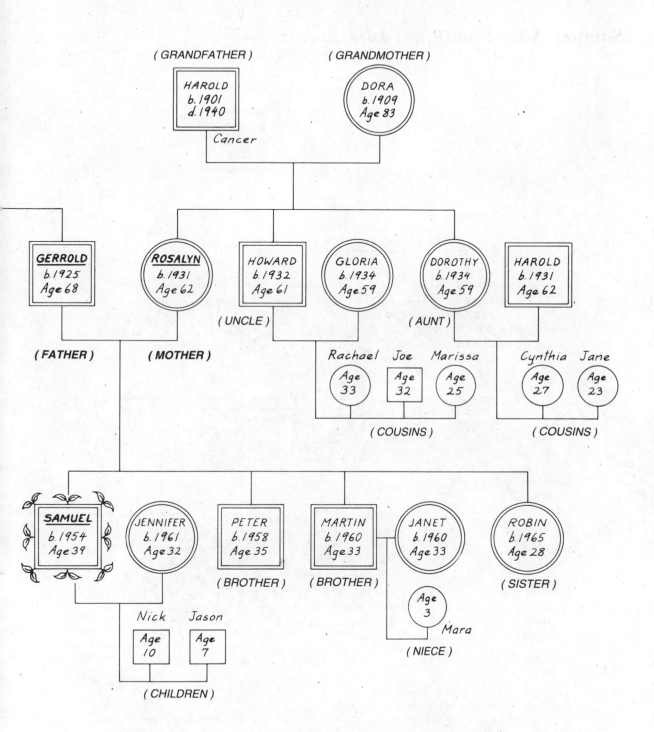

(GRANDFATHER)

HAROLD
b. 1901
d. 1940

Cancer

(GRANDMOTHER)

DORA
b. 1909
Age 83

GERROLD
b. 1925
Age 68

(FATHER)

ROSALYN
b. 1931
Age 62

(MOTHER)

HOWARD
b. 1932
Age 61

(UNCLE)

GLORIA
b. 1934
Age 59

DOROTHY
b. 1934
Age 59

(AUNT)

HAROLD
b. 1931
Age 62

Rachael
Age 33

Joe
Age 32

Marissa
Age 25

(COUSINS)

Cynthia
Age 27

Jane
Age 23

(COUSINS)

SAMUEL
b. 1954
Age 39

JENNIFER
b. 1961
Age 32

PETER
b. 1958
Age 35

(BROTHER)

MARTIN
b. 1960
Age 33

(BROTHER)

JANET
b. 1960
Age 33

ROBIN
b. 1965
Age 28

(SISTER)

Nick
Age 10

Jason
Age 7

(CHILDREN)

Age 3

Mara

(NIECE)

Samuel Adds Significant Life Events

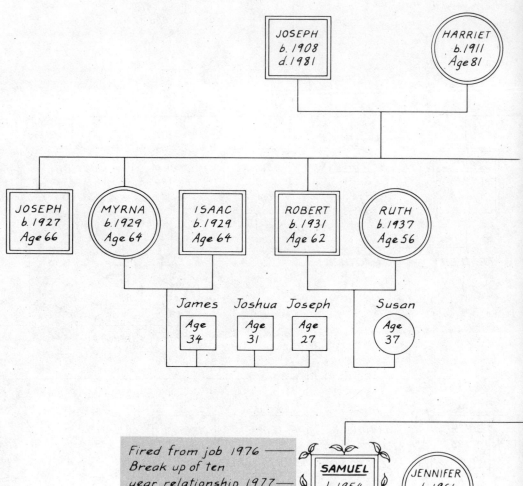

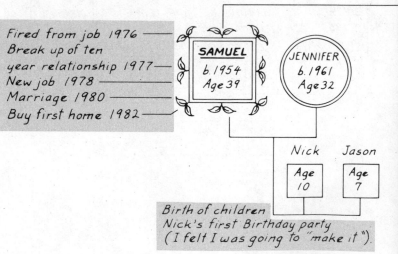

Fired from job 1976 ———
Break up of ten
year relationship 1977 ———
New job 1978 ———
Marriage 1980 ———
Buy first home 1982 ———

Birth of children
Nick's first Birthday party
(I felt I was going to "make it")

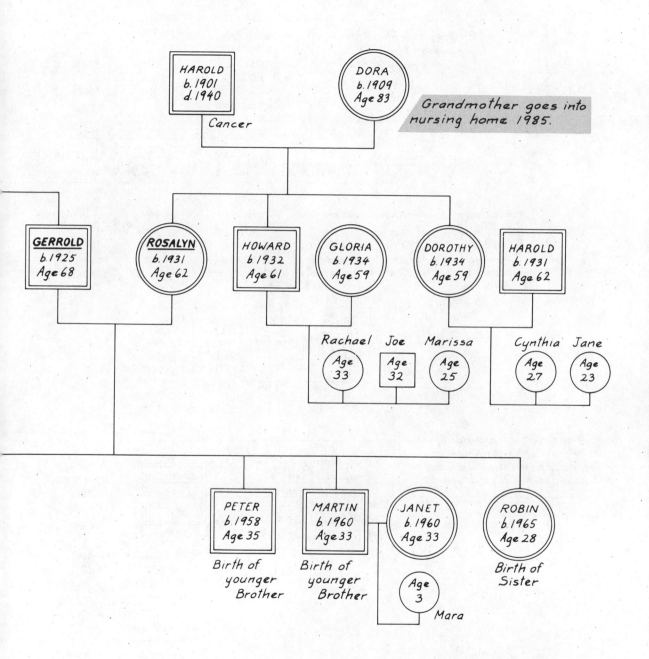

HAROLD
b.1901
d.1940

Cancer

DORA
b.1909
Age 83

Grandmother goes into
nursing home 1985.

GERROLD
b.1925
Age 68

ROSALYN
b.1931
Age 62

HOWARD
b.1932
Age 61

GLORIA
b.1934
Age 59

DOROTHY
b.1934
Age 59

HAROLD
b.1931
Age 62

Rachael
Age 33

Joe
Age 32

Marissa
Age 25

Cynthia
Age 27

Jane
Age 23

PETER
b.1958
Age 35

MARTIN
b.1960
Age 33

JANET
b.1960
Age 33

ROBIN
b.1965
Age 28

Birth of
younger
Brother

Birth of
younger
Brother

Age
3

Mara

Birth of
Sister

Samuel Adds Physical, Mental, and Emotional Issues

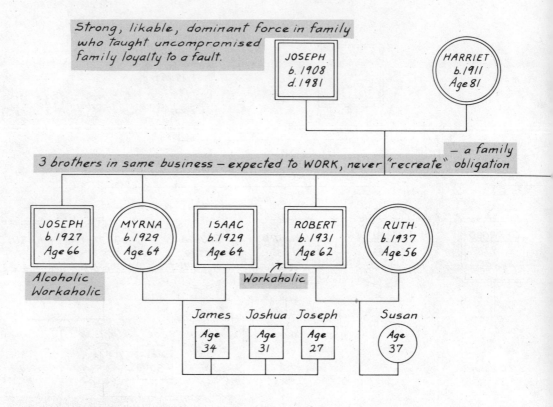

Strong, likable, dominant force in family who taught uncompromised family loyalty to a fault.

JOSEPH
b. 1908
d. 1981

HARRIET
b. 1911
Age 81

3 brothers in same business — expected to WORK, never "recreate" — a family obligation

JOSEPH
b. 1927
Age 66

MYRNA
b. 1929
Age 64

ISAAC
b. 1929
Age 64

ROBERT
b. 1931
Age 62

RUTH
b. 1937
Age 56

Alcoholic
Workaholic

Workaholic

James
Age 34

Joshua
Age 31

Joseph
Age 27

Susan
Age 37

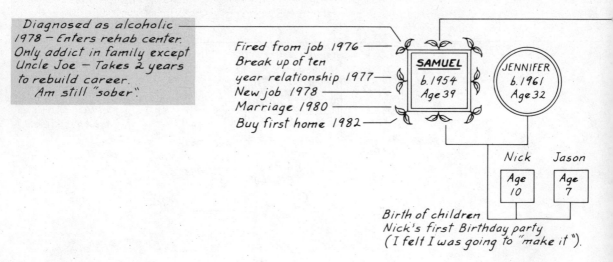

Diagnosed as alcoholic 1978 — Enters rehab center. Only addict in family except Uncle Joe — Takes 2 years to rebuild career. Am still "sober".

Fired from job 1976
Break up of ten year relationship 1977
New job 1978
Marriage 1980
Buy first home 1982

SAMUEL
b. 1954
Age 39

JENNIFER
b. 1961
Age 32

Nick
Age 10

Jason
Age 7

Birth of children
Nick's first Birthday party
(I felt I was going to "make it").

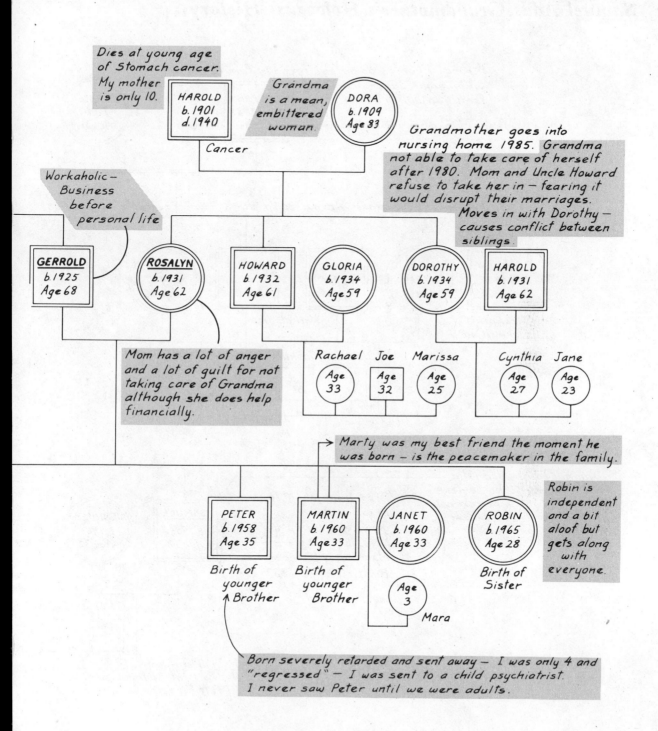

Dies at young age
of Stomach cancer.
My mother
is only 10.

HAROLD
b. 1901
d. 1940

Cancer

Grandma
is a mean,
embittered
woman.

DORA
b. 1909
Age 83

Grandmother goes into
nursing home 1985. Grandma
not able to take care of herself
after 1980. Mom and Uncle Howard
refuse to take her in — fearing it
would disrupt their marriages.
    Moves in with Dorothy —
causes conflict between
siblings.

Workaholic —
Business
before
personal life

GERROLD
b. 1925
Age 68

ROSALYN
b. 1931
Age 62

HOWARD
b. 1932
Age 61

GLORIA
b. 1934
Age 59

DOROTHY
b. 1934
Age 59

HAROLD
b. 1931
Age 62

Mom has a lot of anger
and a lot of guilt for not
taking care of Grandma
although she does help
financially.

Rachael   Joe   Marissa

Age
33

Age
32

Age
25

Cynthia   Jane

Age
27

Age
23

Marty was my best friend the moment he
was born — is the peacemaker in the family.

Robin is
independent
and a bit
aloof but
gets along
with
everyone.

PETER
b. 1958
Age 35

MARTIN
b. 1960
Age 33

JANET
b. 1960
Age 33

ROBIN
b. 1965
Age 28

Birth of
younger
↑ Brother

Birth of
younger
Brother

Age
3

Mara

Birth of
Sister

Born severely retarded and sent away — I was only 4 and
"regressed" — I was sent to a child psychiatrist.
I never saw Peter until we were adults.

Samuel Adds Grandmother's Holocaust History

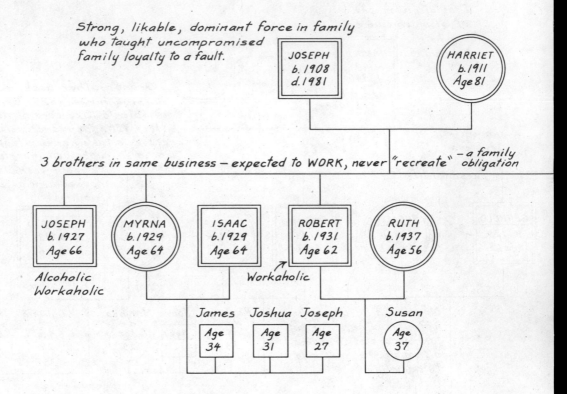

Strong, likable, dominant force in family
who taught uncompromised
family loyalty to a fault.

JOSEPH
b. 1908
d. 1981

HARRIET
b. 1911
Age 81

3 brothers in same business — expected to WORK, never "recreate" — a family obligation

JOSEPH
b. 1927
Age 66

MYRNA
b. 1929
Age 64

ISAAC
b. 1929
Age 64

ROBERT
b. 1931
Age 62

RUTH
b. 1937
Age 56

Alcoholic
Workaholic

Workaholic

James   Joshua   Joseph   Susan

Age 34   Age 31   Age 27   Age 37

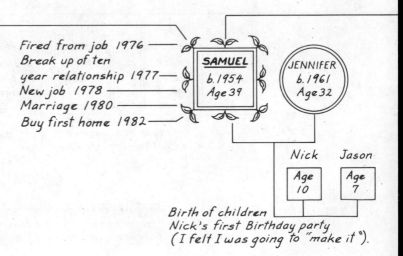

Diagnosed as alcoholic
1978 — Enters rehab center.
Only addict in family except
Uncle Joe — Takes 2 years
to rebuild career.
   Am still "sober".

Fired from job 1976
Break up of ten
year relationship 1977
New job 1978
Marriage 1980
Buy first home 1982

SAMUEL
b. 1954
Age 39

JENNIFER
b. 1961
Age 32

Nick   Jason

Age 10   Age 7

Birth of children
Nick's first Birthday party
(I felt I was going to "make it").

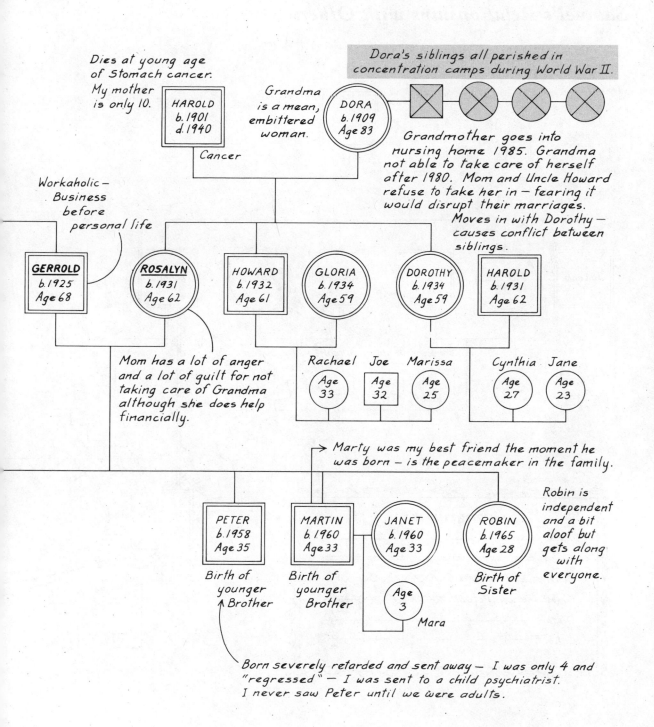

Dies at young age
of Stomach cancer.
My mother
is only 10.

HAROLD
b. 1901
d. 1940

Grandma
is a mean,
embittered
woman.

DORA
b. 1909
Age 83

Dora's siblings all perished in
concentration camps during World War II.

Cancer

Grandmother goes into
nursing home 1985. Grandma
not able to take care of herself
after 1980. Mom and Uncle Howard
refuse to take her in — fearing it
would disrupt their marriages.
Moves in with Dorothy —
causes conflict between
siblings.

Workaholic —
Business
before
personal life

GERROLD
b. 1925
Age 68

ROSALYN
b. 1931
Age 62

HOWARD
b. 1932
Age 61

GLORIA
b. 1934
Age 59

DOROTHY
b. 1934
Age 59

HAROLD
b. 1931
Age 62

Mom has a lot of anger
and a lot of guilt for not
taking care of Grandma
although she does help
financially.

Rachael
Age
33

Joe
Age
32

Marissa
Age
25

Cynthia
Age
27

Jane
Age
23

Marty was my best friend the moment he
was born — is the peacemaker in the family.

Robin is
independent
and a bit
aloof but
gets along
with
everyone.

PETER
b. 1958
Age 35

MARTIN
b. 1960
Age 33

JANET
b. 1960
Age 33

ROBIN
b. 1965
Age 28

Age
3

Mara

Birth of
younger
Brother

Birth of
younger
Brother

Birth of
Sister

Born severely retarded and sent away — I was only 4 and
"regressed" — I was sent to a child psychiatrist.
I never saw Peter until we were adults.

Samuel's Relationships with Others

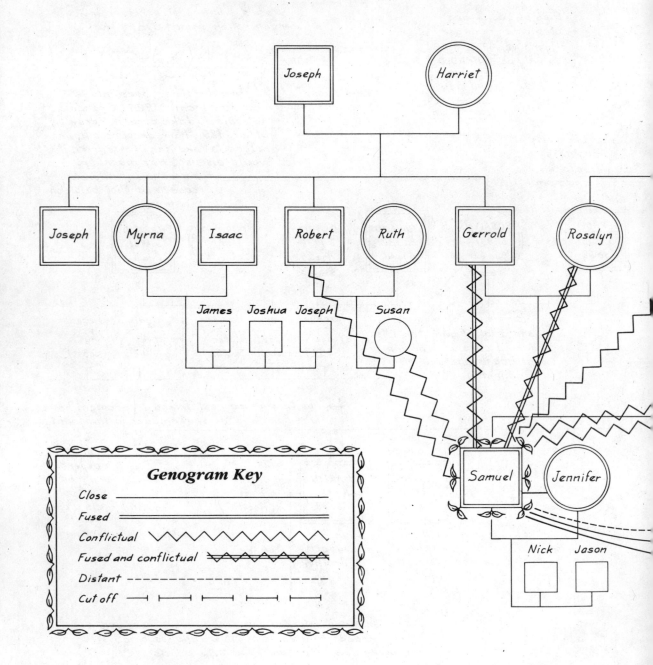

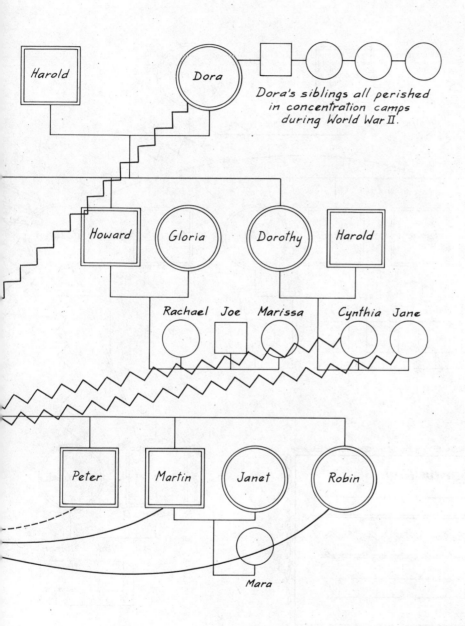

Harold

Dora

*Dora's siblings all perished
in concentration camps
during World War II.*

Howard   Gloria   Dorothy   Harold

Rachael   Joe   Marissa   Cynthia   Jane

Peter   Martin   Janet   Robin

Mara

Samuel's Mother's Relationships with Others Important in Her Life

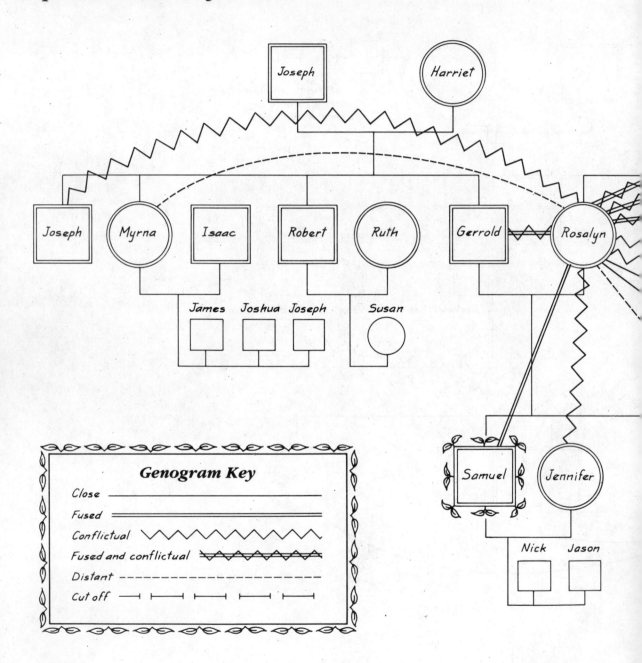

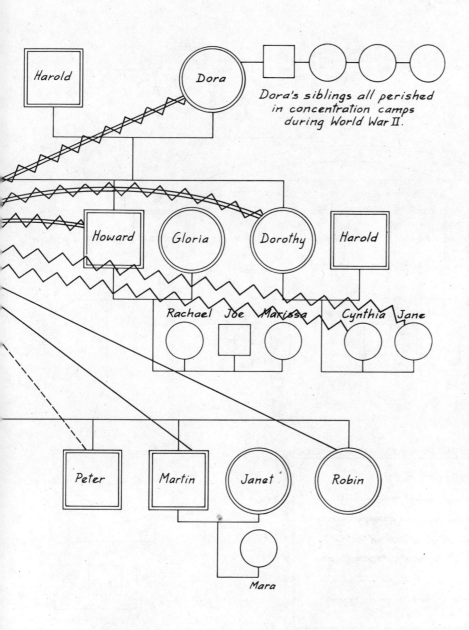

Harold

Dora

Dora's siblings all perished
in concentration camps
during World War II.

Howard   Gloria   Dorothy   Harold

Rachael   Joe   Marissa   Cynthia   Jane

Peter   Martin   Janet   Robin

Mara

Samuel's Father's Relationships with Others Important in His Life

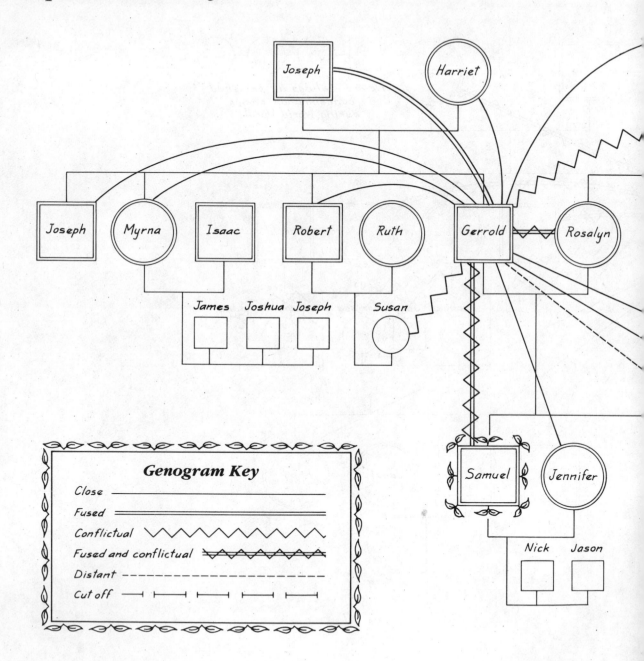

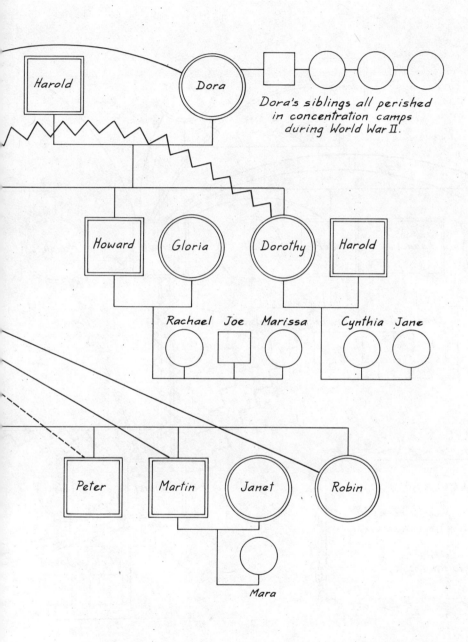

Dora's siblings all perished
in concentration camps
during World War II.

Finished Genogram (Filled with Closeness and Conflict)

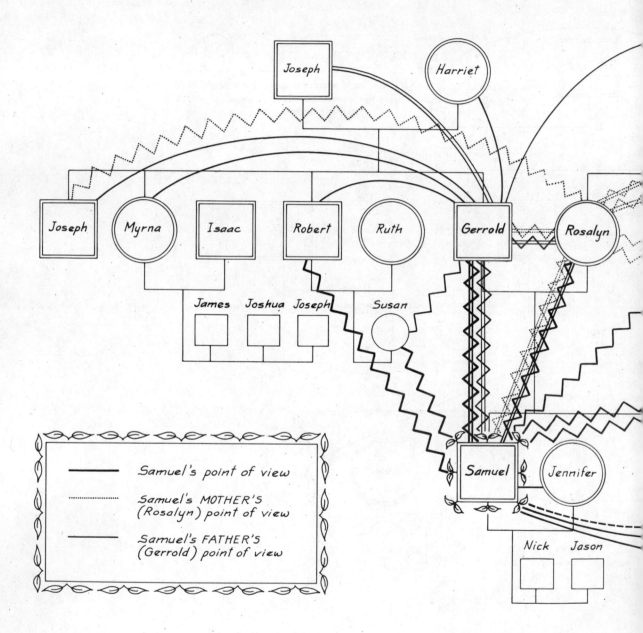

Legend:

——————— Samuel's point of view

·············· Samuel's MOTHER'S (Rosalyn) point of view

——————— Samuel's FATHER'S (Gerrold) point of view

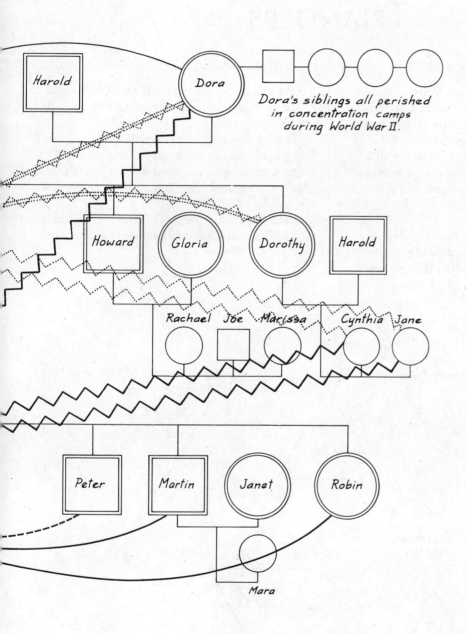

Harold

Dora

*Dora's siblings all perished
in concentration camps
during World War II.*

Howard

Gloria

Dorothy

Harold

Rachael Joe Marissa Cynthia Jane

Peter

Martin

Janet

Robin

Mara

TRIANGLES

amily therapist Murray Bowen developed the concept of "triangles" to illustrate how family members react to each other. Bowen believed that two-person relationships are often shaky, and the two will often draw in a third person as a stabilizer. Sometimes one person will bring in another so he or she will have an ally, and it becomes two against one.

Bowen further believed that the degree to which a person becomes emotionally mature is based less on how others in the triangle might react and more on personal needs and values.

Are you involved in such a triangle? Are there other triangles in your family?

Samuel looked at his family groupings and began to identify important triangles. He illustrated them with the same symbolic lines used on his genogram. As a reminder, here are those symbols:

Let's see how Samuel's primary "triangle" (with his mother and father) looks on his genogram.

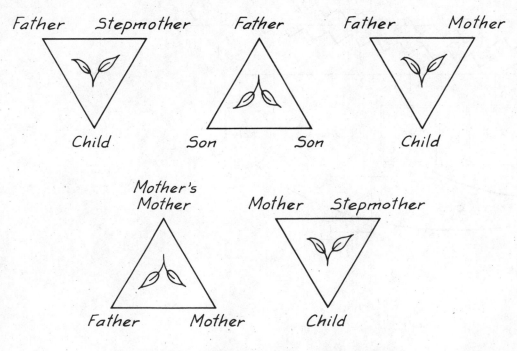

Examples of Common Triangles

Samuel's Triangles
Triangle with Parents:

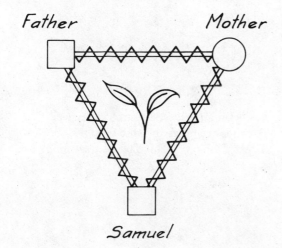

I often felt my mom spoke for my dad, that she could control the triangle. If I spoke with my dad directly, there would be a different outcome; more melodramatic, sometimes more anger, but with a more honest resolution. But my mom was the one who did the controlling—she's still trying to do that.

Triangle with Parents and Brother Marty:

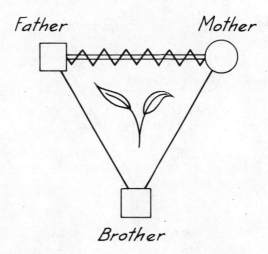

Mom, Dad, and Marty are all close. Marty visits them with his wife and kids all the time. In a way, it gets me off the hook. I couldn't stand to be with them as much as he is. He is living up to my father's expectations of family closeness, and he plays into my mother's love of control.

Triangle with Me, Mom, and Grandma Dora:

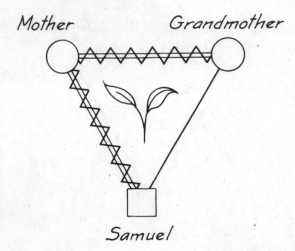

My grandmother Dora, Mom's mother, always treated me like a prince, so I should feel very close to her, and in some ways I do. But I'm angry at the way she has treated my mother. They were never able to communicate without some degree of tension. When my grandmother became ill, she felt guilty for becoming so dependent, and my mother felt guilty for not agreeing to let her live with us. As a young widow, my grandmother worked very hard for years to raise her children, but didn't offer emotional support and was bitter and abusive. I have problems separating myself from what they have done to each other. I don't know how to draw the lines of this triangle.

Triangle with Me, Mom, and Jennifer (My Wife):

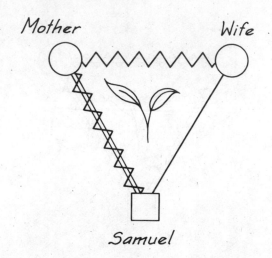

Jennifer is always encouraging me to separate from the anger and guilt my mother uses on me. This is frustrating for Mom, because she is always asking me to translate Jennifer's behavior to her. She is clearly displeased with the influence Jennifer has over me, and that makes me angry. I should be able to make my own decisions.

Triangle with Mom, Dad, and Grandma Dora:

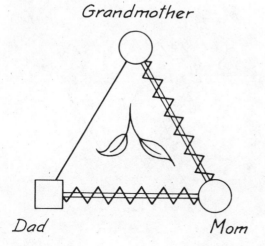

Dad often referees their conflicts. He has tried to smooth out my mother's anger toward Grandma. Her anger is a result of being so emotionally abused and constantly criticized by Grandma.

"You are now ready for the final step in filling out the genogram," Mauksch told Samuel. "Ask those same questions from your parents' perspective. What was it like for your mother or father to be in your triangle or in triangles with other members of the family? Does this help you understand how they became who they are? Describe the triangles your parents would think are important." Samuel completed the following triangles:

Triangles from His Parents' Point of View
Triangle with Mom, Dad, and Me:

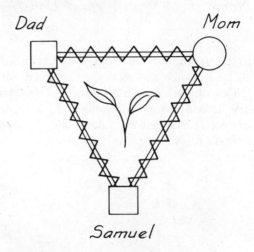

For my mom, I guess this triangle has been equally frustrating and rewarding. Dad always played devil's advocate with her. She felt he was fair almost to a fault, and so did I. It's as if he couldn't or wouldn't get emotionally involved. I'm more larcenous than my dad so my mother never knew what to expect from me. For Dad, he seems conflicted between our triangle and his own family. He had a softer spot than my mom and seems to have found the triangle more rewarding, seeing life with me as unpredictable, but accepting me more. Still, it's frustrating for him because he believes so strongly in a tightly knit family, and I don't fit into that.

Triangle with Mom, Her Mother (Dora), and My Aunt Dorothy:

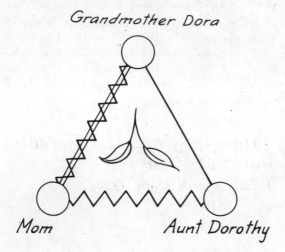

This has been tough for Mom. She feels tension with her mother and feels she can't live with her. Dorothy is close with Grandma Dora, but angry at Mom for "dumping" Dora at her doorstep. It changed the relationship between the sisters forever.

Triangle with Mom, Me, and Jennifer:

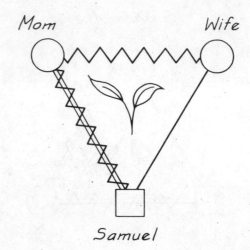

Mom seems jealous that Jennifer has more influence over me than she does. I guess it hurts her in the same way it hurts her that Dad's brothers have so much influence over Dad.

Triangle with Dad, Robert, and Joseph:

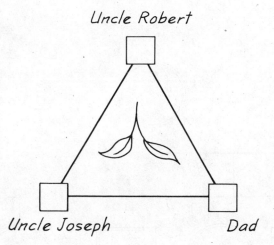

These three brothers are bonded with super-glue, fused at the hip (or should I say wallet?). They are in business together, and all expect a great deal from each other. There is a lot of pressure, but they have all found a way to get along. Dad has always been torn between this fraternal triangle and Mom and the kids, but it seems that this triangle usually wins out.

Triangle with Dad, Mom, and Uncle Robert:

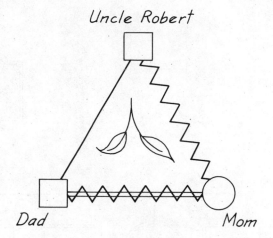

Uncle Robert and my dad are the closest of his siblings, and to my mother, Robert represents Dad's obsession with the business, so she had a great deal of antagonism toward Robert. She feels Robert has pulled Dad away from her and our family.

From my dad's perspective, he just tries to keep the peace but clearly expects Mom to accept his closeness with his brother, and doesn't think there needs to be a conflict. But he clearly feels the pressure from Mom, so there is tension.

How a Triangle Looks on a Genogram

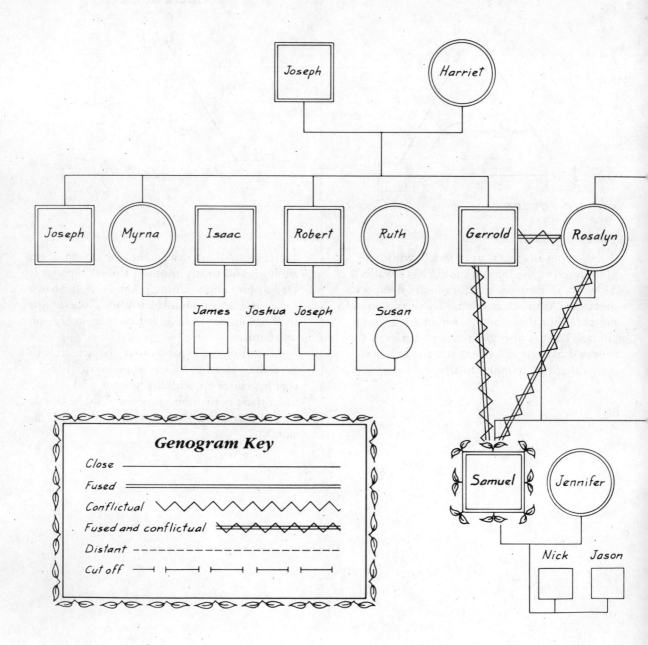

Genogram Key

Close ——————————————
Fused ════════════════
Conflictual ∿∿∿∿∿∿∿∿∿
Fused and conflictual ⨉⨉⨉⨉⨉⨉
Distant – – – – – – – – –
Cut off —|—|———|——|———|——|—

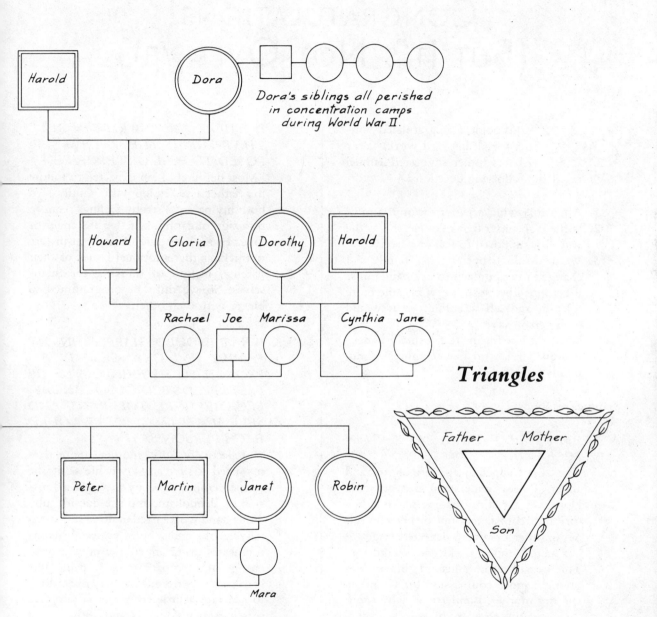

Dora's siblings all perished
in concentration camps
during World War II.

Triangles

CONGRATULATIONS!
(BUT IT'S NOT OVER YET)

At this point, I congratulated Samuel for all his hard work. Larry Mauksch then suggested Samuel ask himself the following questions:

1. Am I following a pattern in my family?
2. Is there an unwritten rule that this is the way I'm supposed to feel or perceive?
3. What would happen in my family if I changed my approach to my painpoints? If I stopped being so angry, became more tolerant and self-accepting, what would each person say?
4. What's it like for me to try small changes in how I relate to key members of my family?

Samuel responds:

1. *AM I FOLLOWING A PATTERN IN MY FAMILY?*
"Yes, I'm trapped in a pattern of guilt and anger. I now understand my grandma Dora was a victim of some horrible historical circumstances out of her control. My mother became a deflected target of her anger, and it trickled down to me. This doesn't change history, but it does give me more compassion for Grandma and my mother. I understand why Mom is so sensitive to everything.

"On my father's side, I see that family is everything. He and his brothers selfishly guard their position in the business as well as the family, almost as if it's a sign of caring. To slack off or leave the business would symbolize a lack of love."

2. *IS THERE AN UNWRITTEN RULE THAT THIS IS THE WAY I'M SUPPOSED TO FEEL OR PERCEIVE?*
"Most definitely I am expected to follow my father's obsession with family. To both my parents, strong feelings seem to be a sign of caring, whether it's anger or love. I see that some of my cousins are mimicking the emotional issues of their parents, instead of thinking for themselves. So we must be programmed to bicker with each other."

3. *WHAT WOULD HAPPEN IN MY FAMILY IF I CHANGED MY APPROACH TO MY PAINPOINTS? (IF I STOPPED BEING SO ANGRY, BECAME MORE TOLERANT AND SELF-ACCEPTING, WHAT WOULD EACH PERSON SAY?*
"Intellectually, my mother appreciates my need to live my own life. But she seemed embarrassed by my open admission of alcoholism, and she doesn't fully understand what I need to do to stay mentally healthy and sober. Because she communicates using anger, the only way to change my approach to these painpoints is to separate more from her. But if I try to separate a little from the family, she sees it as abandonment and selfishness. I wonder if it has something to do with her father dying young or my dad often putting the business before her.

"My dad would react better than my mom if I stayed out of my family's angry and intolerant communication. After all, he tries to be the peacemaker. He'll say 'do what you want to do' but I always feel a tinge of guilt attached. But because he never has emotionally invested in me, he would be more accepting if I change my relationship with the family."

4. *WHAT'S IT LIKE FOR ME TO TRY SMALL CHANGES IN HOW I RELATE TO KEY MEMBERS OF MY FAMILY?*
"With my wife's encouragement, I have already begun to separate from these family patterns. I'm starting to say no to my family. But they think I'm being selfish, and they take the separation personally, as if I don't love them anymore. But it is the only way to calm my anger, the overwhelming conflict in my genogram. I realize I can't *change* the family pattern. I still struggle with separating, and sometimes hate myself for being a spineless wimp when it comes to my family."

Mauksch suggested that Samuel try not to analyze this alone. "Choose someone you trust—your wife or a close friend, perhaps. Find someone to talk to, to help you have a clear head when you analyze your genogram. Listen to yourself as you talk about it."

"I can hardly believe this," Samuel told me days later. "I learned more from this exercise then my last four years of therapy." This comment will no doubt annoy some well-trained therapists, but it is a fact that Samuel spent several years with a reputable therapist and never once was his grandmother's pain and anguish over the Holocaust explored. If, after doing a genogram you see disturbing family patterns, be sure to consult a family therapist, a specialty within the field of mental health.

Should You Involve Your Family?

In the middle of this whole process, Samuel asked Larry Mauksch if he could get help from other family members in answering some of the genogram questions. "Fill it out yourself first,"

Mauksch answered. "If you find you are curious to know more, then you could go to the people in your family. But be cautious how you ask." Mauksch suggested guidelines for asking family members potentially emotional questions:

1. The reason to talk to other family members is to better understand their view of the world, how their experiences affected the way they handled their relationships with you.
2. Set your issues aside. Make sure your general anger and blame do not spill over in your questions—otherwise, your questions won't be productive.
3. You should feel some comfort with the people you choose to question. Be sensitive to what their reactions might be, and be especially aware of any possible effects your questions may have on their health.
4. It is not a good idea to speak with someone you fiercely blame for something, or with whom you are so angry you cannot be objective.

Sample Questions for Family Members Using These Guidelines

1. To a parent
   WRONG: "What did you do to make me so screwed up?" (This is a *blaming* statement.)
   RIGHT: "What was it like to be a parent? What decisions did you make about parenting and how did you arrive at those decisions?" (This is a question from *their* point of view.)

2. To a father
   WRONG: "Why did you mistreat Mother?" (Again, this is a *blaming* statement.)
   RIGHT: "What was it like being in a relationship with Mom?" (This could open up a whole new world of understanding your father's point of view.)

Finding Family Strengths: The Other Way to Interpret Your Genogram

While Samuel might look at his genogram and worry about its mixed messages, he can also celebrate its strengths. Here's just some of what can give him courage in his life:

1. His grandmother Dora may be an embittered woman, but she is a survivor in the purest sense. Losing one's family to the Holocaust must have been an almost unendurable devastation. Yet Dora kept on going, raised a family, and is enjoying her grandchildren.
2. His mother might feel guilty for not having taken Dora into her home, but she is clearly a woman who knows her limits and has the courage to let others know. She seems to be willing to live with the consequences of her decisions.
3. Perhaps the greatest strength in Samuel's genogram is the closeness of his father's family. Although it might seem suffocating at times, they appear to be loyal and uncompromising in their belief that family comes first. Samuel needs to learn to enjoy this rich heritage, yet learn from his mother how to set limits.

4. Samuel's immediate family, his wife and children, appear to be an oasis in a troubled landscape. He can draw strength from them.

What Does It All Mean?

Samuel sees a pattern of strained and bitter relationships on his mother's side. At the root of his bitterness was his grandmother's tragic loss of her family in the Holocaust.

Samuel sees on his father's side a smothering closeness. His father expects him to experience the same closeness and will not tolerate anything less.

So from Samuel's genogram we see he is torn between two messages: one that says family is a source of pain and anger, the other that family is a source of total strength and unchallenged loyalty. This helps to explain Samuel's painpoints: *anger* from his mother's side, and *intolerance* from his father's side. This leaves Samuel confused about his own values: No matter how he behaves, he has trouble accepting himself (his third painpoint: *lack of self-acceptance.*)

Using the genogram, Samuel was able to find subtle (and not-so-subtle) patterns that

ARE DIVORCES CAUSED BY GENES?

*T*his once ludicrous statement has been given new life, thanks to a study at the University of Minnesota.

The study looked at 1,500 middle-aged twins (half identical, half fraternal) and found the divorce rate significantly higher for identical twins whose other twin divorced.

In this study, the overall divorce rate was 20 percent. But the rate rose to 30 percent for those whose fraternal twin divorced (remember that fraternal twins share, on average, half

each other's genes) and rose to 45 percent if the identical twin divorced. Identical twins share the same genes.

Researchers theorize that inherited personality traits are to blame for the sibling similarities. Adults most likely to divorce show anxious, hostile, and strongly assertive behavior. So it stands to reason that if one twin has such characteristics, the other twin is likely to have many of the same personality traits.

programmed him to make certain responses to life's ebb and flow. Much like the genes that predispose us to a certain illness, Samuel was handed family patterns that predisposed him to anger and intolerance in certain situations. Recognizing these patterns has relieved him of his perfectionist guilt and has provided him with a specific goal: to short-circuit these patterns for his own children and not to expect miracles for himself.

"I know that anger is okay," Samuel told me after completing his genogram. "It's simply the way my family communicated. The important thing for me is to realize why it's there, to try and manage it, and to constantly examine my motives."

Genograms for Seriously Troubled Families

Samuel's challenge was to find hidden patterns in a childhood that seemed on the surface to be perfectly stable and happy. Another friend of mine, now in her thirties, has recently been working to understand a far more troubled childhood. For years she and her other siblings were victims of physical and sexual abuse at the hands of their father. After years of hard work with a good therapist, Sarah decided to go to school to become a therapist herself. One of her family therapy classes required her to construct a genogram.

Sarah was kind enough to share that genogram with me, although we have eliminated names to protect her family's privacy. But instead of sticking to the textbook approach, she developed codes that illuminated specific problems. She already knew there was a horrible history in her immediate family: sexual, physical, and verbal abuse, eating disorders, and alcohol and nicotine addiction. She decided to look for those specific painpoints on the lines of her family tree.

"I was concerned about how I was going to get information with all the secrets in my family. And I wondered how they were going to respond," Sarah told me. "I wrote letters to everyone, even my parents. I made them blank charts and asked them nicely to fill them out, not letting them know I was looking for anything specific.

"My father was surprisingly cooperative, and filled out some of the chart from memory. My mother called her sister and they worked on it together. But then I found out that my parents told completely different stories about some things. And other relatives supplied me with only bits and pieces. So I kept pursuing it, talking to cousins, aunts, and uncles.

"Eventually I got a patchwork of stuff that began to make sense. Although others in my class had much more information, I focused on what might have led my father to be so emotionally sick . . . and what would have led my mother to ignore what was going on. I learned that both my father and my mother had been sexually assaulted as children. For my mother, that meant tremendous guilt and denial because of her strict religious upbringing."

Sarah's experience shows that even in cases of absolute horror, a genogram can bring comfort and understanding. "I remember sitting there and saying, 'Oh my God!' It's no wonder. It all made sense to me. Abuse all over the place, alcoholism, family scandals, tragedies, and hatred mixed with strict religious values.

"Emotionally, I became sad. The genogram looked like a real mess. I discussed it with a therapist. I hate what happened to me as a child, but I don't hate my parents anymore. I feel sad they led such hideous lives. The genogram gave me an understanding of where I came from and why everything happened. It helped me move on. My parents are still feeling torment, but now I'm on the other side."

Sarah protected herself from her explosive past by consulting with a therapist while she did the genogram. But she had the curiosity and innovation to target certain secrets in her family. She actually unearthed sexual abuse a few generations back, a remarkable discovery. Finding this one case convinces her there are probably more.

So a genogram can be made to fit your needs and curiosities. While a mental health professional might feel compelled to stick to a more conventional format, you are free to explore

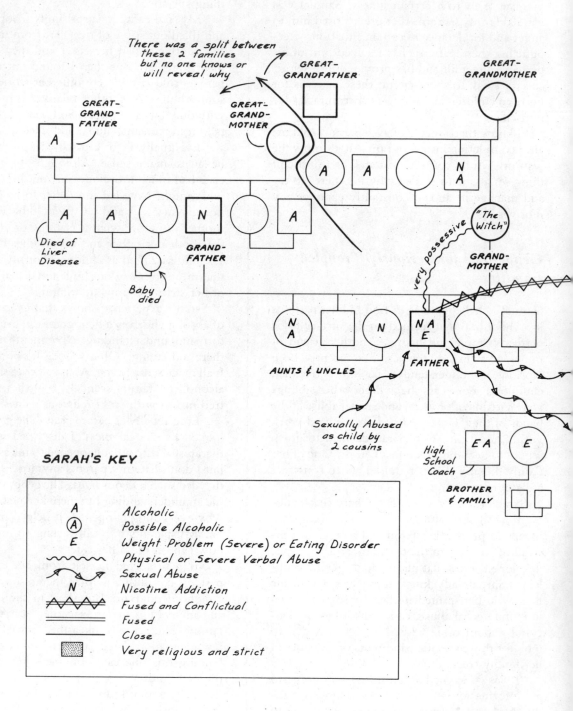

SARAH'S KEY

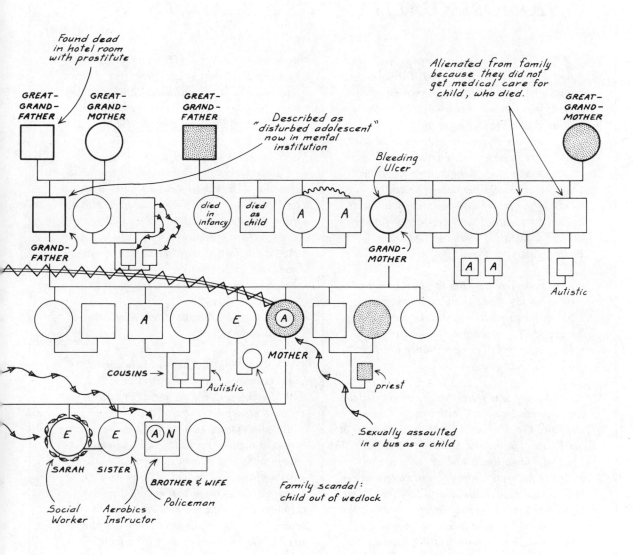

Found dead in hotel room with prostitute

GREAT-GRAND-FATHER

GREAT-GRAND-MOTHER

GREAT-GRAND-FATHER

Described as "disturbed adolescent" now in mental institution

Alienated from family because they did not get medical care for child, who died.

GREAT-GRAND-MOTHER

Bleeding Ulcer

GRAND-FATHER

died in infancy

died as child

A   A

GRAND-MOTHER

A   A

Autistic

A   E   A

priest

COUSINS →

Autistic

MOTHER

Sexually assaulted in a bus as a child

E   E   A N

SARAH   SISTER   BROTHER & WIFE

Social Worker   Aerobics Instructor   Policeman

Family scandal: child out of wedlock

HOMOSEXUALITY: "IT'S A BRAIN THING"

That claim now adorns a popular T-shirt sold in West Hollywood, California—a community with a large homosexual population. It was created after a series of studies concluded that there is a genetic factor that may predispose some men to be gay. In other words, that homosexuality is innate.

One major study done by two researchers (one gay and one heterosexual) recently looked at the rates of homosexuality in identical and nonidentical twin brothers of gay men, as well as adoptive brothers of gay men. Here's what they found:

- *Fifty-two percent of the identical twin brothers were gay (they share the same genes).*
- *Twenty-two percent of nonidentical twins were gay (they share half the same genes).*
- *Eleven percent of the genetically unrelated brothers were gay.*

The study was researched by Michael Bailey, a psychologist at Northwestern University, and Dr. Richard Pillard, a psychiatrist at the Boston University School of Medicine.

At the same time, another study of the brains of forty-one cadavers, including nineteen homosexual men, found that a tiny part of the brain that controls sexual activity was half the size in gay men than it was in heterosexual men (research by neuroscientist Simon Le Vay at the Salk Institute in La Jolla, California).

Another cadaver study, this one at UCLA, shows another physical, inborn difference. Neuroscientists Roger Gorski and Laura Allen found that an important structure connecting the left and right sides of the brain is actually larger in size in gay men (it is already known to be larger in women). Studies done on ca-

davers use primarily AIDS patients, because in many cases their sexual preference is clearly stated on the death certificate. Similar studies have not been done on lesbians after death. But another recent study by the Bailey/Pillard team, this one on lesbians with twin sisters, does suggest a genetic link.

They looked at one hundred fifteen homosexual or bisexual women, all twins with sisters. The one hundred fifteen women also had thirty-two adopted sisters. Their findings:

- *About one in two identical twins were homosexual or bisexual.*
- *one in six fraternal twins were homosexual or bisexual.*
- *one in sixteen adoptive sisters were homosexual or bisexual.*

These findings are significant because if homosexuality were strictly environmental, then lesbianism would be just as prevalent among the adoptive sisters.

But as evidence mounts that homosexuality may be a matter of genetics, not "parenting" or environmental influences, some gay activists are not pleased. If, indeed, a "gay gene" is found, does that mean that eventually homosexuality can be altered in utero? And do gays need a biological explanation to be accepted? Are they to be tolerated only if they are "born that way"?

This criticism surprises the researchers who did the twin studies on men. They argue that a biological foundation would discourage claims that homosexuals can "recruit" heterosexuals.

While the political debate goes on, scientists are likely to continue their quest for a "gay gene."

and experiment. But if the work starts to sting emotionally, and you feel uncomfortable, by all means continue the genogram, but under the guidance of a therapist.

For Samuel and Sarah, seeing their past on a chart was oddly comforting. "The craziness is going to stop—on my line of the chart at least," Sarah told me, "and that alone was worth the work."

Learn to Decode Your Behavioral Family Tree

What can we learn from Sarah's behavioral family tree? She began with almost a blank slate, focusing on sexual abuse. But she knew from her training as a social worker that sexually deviant behavior is often linked to other behavioral disorders or dysfunction in families. She focused on other problems she saw in her immediate family—alcoholism, eating disorders, and family conflict—to see how far back such behavior went in her family chain.

As she began to unearth family "secrets," she became more specific in her focus. It was difficult to trace eating disorders back more than one generation, possibly because it was an undefined condition until recent years. But she found definite evidence of physical and sexual abuse, as well as overly dramatic conflicts, including a serious family dispute over poor medical care for an autistic child.

As you set out to do your family genogram (Your Own Genogram Workbook begins on page 147) remember that it might take some twists and turns you didn't anticipate. Sarah didn't know, for example, that her father had been sexually abused by two cousins. It seems impossible that he would have kept this information from her after she confronted him with his crimes, but he was either too ashamed or in complete denial of the depth of his problems.

In fact, Sarah's genogram shows us a pattern of dysfunction so severe that she could better understand why there had been no one to help her father through his experience as a victim of abuse, just as there had been no one with the coping skills to help her. This information was useful to Sarah, not so she could forgive her father (that is not the point here), but so she could understand that his attacks on her were not personal, not aimed at punishing or hurting her, but were instead an angry reaction to his own abuse and neglect as a child.

Let's take a look at a few of Sarah's triangles:

From Sarah's Point of View:

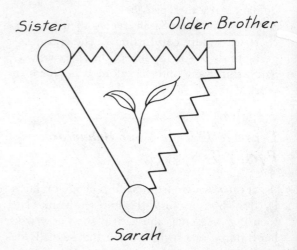

Sarah, her mother, and her father:
Sarah has a conflictual relationship with her mother, and is cut off from her father. But her parents' relationship is "fused and conflictual." They are divorced, but because they still see each other and are still close, this remains a difficult situation for Sarah.

Sarah, her sister, and their older brother:
Sarah and her sister (who was not sexually abused) are very close. They have both been in therapy and acknowledge the serious problems in the family. But their older brother (also not sexually abused) refuses to accept his father's behavior and views Sarah as the troublemaker. The brother's relationship with both sisters is conflictual.

Like Samuel, Sarah also completed triangles from her parents' perspectives.

From Her Father's Point of View:

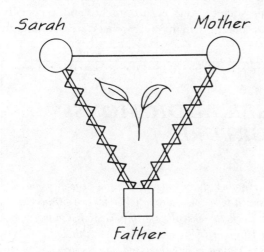

Sarah, her father, and her mother:
Her father admits his abuse, but denies its overwhelming impact on the family. Hence, he would view this triangle differently, seeing himself as fused and conflicted with Sarah, and seeing Sarah and her mother as close.

From Her Mother's Point of View:

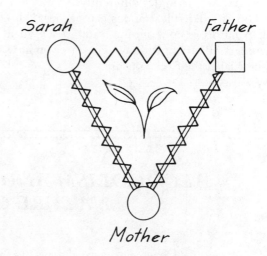

Sarah, her mother, and her father:
Her mother has confusion all the way around. She would see herself as fused and conflicted with both Sarah and her ex-husband, and she'd recognize that Sarah and her father are now mostly estranged.

Note how everyone in Sarah's primary triangle (Sarah, her mother, and her father) would interpret their triangles differently.

This is where illustrations can be very helpful. A family is not communicating well when members of a triangle don't even agree on how to best label their relationship.

You Mean I Was Born This Way?

Sarah's genogram might look exceptional, unusual, over-the-edge. But it is a living document that supports the newest trends in research. As we decompress from a century of Freudian belief that our behavior is caused by our society, our environment, and especially our parents, many researchers are looking to

---

ALCOHOLISM AND OTHER ADDICTIONS: NATURE OR NURTURE?

It has long been noted that addictions like alcoholism run in families. But are children learning addiction from their parents' behavior, or do they inherit a predisposition?

A well-known study in Denmark followed the lives of 5,500 people adopted at an early age. It revealed that the biological sons of alcoholics were more than three times as likely to become alcoholics than the biological sons of nonalcoholics—even when they were raised in nonalcoholic homes.

Some researchers in California recently claimed they had found at least one of the genetic factors in alcoholism. A study published in the October 1991 Journal of the American Medical Association says a gene found in blood and tissue samples appears to be more prevalent not only in alcoholics but in behavioral disorders like autism, attention deficit disorder (hyperactivity), Tourette's syndrome (which causes bizarre facial tics and uncontrollable cursing in some patients), and post-traumatic stress disorder. (The study was done by scientists at the City of Hope Medical Center in Duarte.)

This follows a study in the spring of 1990 at UCLA and the University of Texas, which found the gene in 77 percent of people with a severe form of alcoholism.

Another study suggests that the tendency for women to become alcoholics is at least 50 percent genetic. Scientists at the Medical College of Virginia (Virginia Commonwealth University) looked at one thousand pairs of female twins, both identical and fraternal.

They learned that if one twin was alcoholic, the chance the other twin would also be alcoholic was much higher among identical twins compared to fraternal twins (26 percent versus 12 percent, compared to 5 percent in the general population).

These twin studies, plus a possible dopamine or serotonin connection give weight to the theory that substance abuse is strongly hereditary in many cases. While not all studies confirm these findings, the evidence tilts in favor of some kind of genetic theory for severe addictive behavior (with one's upbringing being another factor.) This has spawned an explosion in the field of "neurogenetics," the link between behavior and genes. Think of the possibilities if one day the children of people with compulsive behavior could be tested to see if they have a similar gene! Surely social factors play a part in behavior, but the possibility that there's a genetic component too is a controversial idea that will be discussed more over the next decade.

genetics once again to explain a family history like Sarah's.

A study published in the October 1991 *Journal of the American Medical Association* says a single gene found in blood and tissue samples appears to be more prevalent in people with a variety of behavioral disorders, including substance abuse, depression, and schizophrenia.

This startling claim brought with it the thought-provoking premise that many different behavioral problems could be genetically connected. But more recently, scientists have publicly backed away from this theory, saying it is probably a mixture of several genes that predisposes people to mental illness.

If the single-gene theory had been confirmed, it would have meant that a single treatment, a simple form of gene therapy, might have worked on hundreds of thousands of people with genetically linked behavioral problems. Instead, genetic treatments are further away because it will take time to find interwoven groups of genes.

To make it more complicated, the connection between genetically linked mental illness and environment is still fuzzy. What really pushes one over the edge? A bad gene or a life crisis? Biology or circumstances? When you complete your own genogram, you will learn this is not as important a question as you might think. What really matters in your first step toward emotional peace is recognizing a pattern, whether it be genetic or otherwise.

HOW CAN BEHAVIOR HAVE A BIOLOGICAL CONNECTION?

This is the key question at the root of the nature versus nurture debate. It is now accepted that certain chemicals in our brains are directly linked to behavior. We know this because, after much experimentation, psychiatrists are able to alter, control, and manage some behavioral problems using prescription drugs. If scientists can confirm that these levels are passed on genetically (there is already much evidence to support this), a look at your family behavioral history becomes even more important. There are two chemicals that seem to play the biggest role in human behavior. We have heard about these chemicals in various news reports, but their functions are confusing. These chemicals are dopamine and serotonin. The following is a general summary of how abnormal levels of each may manifest.

DOPAMINE: Regulates motor activity. There are five known diseases directly linked to dopamine abnormalities:

1. Schizophrenia (symptoms include bizarre thoughts, hearing voices, and paranoid behavior).
2. Parkinson's disease (symptoms include trembling, unbalanced posture, shuffling walk).
3. Huntington's chorea (symptoms usually appear after the age of thirty-five and include random twitching and clumsiness, as well as deterioration of mental abilities).
4. Tourette's syndrome (symptoms include bizarre facial tics, barklike sounds, and, in about half the cases, uncontrolled cursing).
5. Attention deficit disorder (symptoms appear early in life and include inattentiveness, impulsive behavior, and sometimes hyperactivity).

All of these dopamine-related problems involve some sort of physical or motor dysfunction, although each one has other unique behavioral symptoms.

SEROTONIN: Called the "great inhibitor" or the "civilizing" brain chemical.

Some researchers believe excessively low serotonin levels may contribute to the following:

1. Aggression
2. Alcoholism
3. Arson
4. Borderline personality disorder (long-term unstable behavior)
5. Bulemia
6. Migraine headaches
7. Premenstrual tension (PMS)
8. Violent behavior
9. Violent suicide
10. Clinical depression

On the other hand, excessively high serotonin levels may contribute to:

1. Autism (symptoms appear within the first year of life; child begins to withdraw from human relationships and usually does not respond to human affection)
2. Infantile spasms
3. Manic-depressive disorder
4. Schizophrenia
5. Some types of mental retardation

When serotonin receptors are hypersensitive, it may result in:

1. Obsessive-compulsive disorder
2. Panic attacks

When doctors artificially stimulate dopamine, or inhibit serotonin, it can result in increased aggression and sexual activity. This further supports the biological/behavioral/connection.

One Theory of How "Dope" Got Its Name

Dopamine is connected to what we commonly call the "pleasure centers" in the brain. It has long been known that addictive drugs, including nicotine, prompt a sudden release of dopamine. This leads to the theory that addicts are self-correcting low levels of dopamine when they take their drugs. Studies done on rats show the desire for pleasure is even more important than food. Some studies show rats choosing drugs over food to the point of starving themselves to death.

For addicts, the dopamine/serotonin combination is a lethal double whammy. Too little of either one can encourage addiction as the body desperately tries to adjust itself. Add to this all the emotional and environmental pain that triggers self-medication, and it is easy to understand why addiction is such an overwhelming scourge in our modern life. It is a pattern of self-destruction that should not be taken lightly if you discover it on your family tree.

Sarah's Genogram Begins to Make More Sense

Could Sarah's genogram reveal patterns caused by low levels of serotonin (a brain neurotrans-

SCHIZOPHRENIA: CLUES FROM SWEDEN

*S*chizophrenia is a general term for a group of mental illnesses characterized by disturbances in thinking, in behavior, and in emotional reactions, sometimes accompanied by bizarre delusions. It is the most common form of psychotic illness, and it affects about one and a half million Americans.

Human geneticist Dr. David Comings (at the City of Hope in Duarte, California) describes schizophrenia as the "granddaddy for studies of genetic behavior." Studies of twins as far back as 1928 show genetic links with this behavioral disorder.

Over the years, several family, twin, and adoption studies confirm that genetic factors play an important part in this difficult disease. This brings us to a remote region just above the Arctic Circle in Sweden. In the seventeenth century, three families migrated there from an area that is now Finland. Today, almost all the people still living in that region (the population is over one hundred) can be traced to those three families, so they make a perfect isolated pedigree for study.

Swedish researchers have been studying these people for decades, and currently have pinpointed at least thirty-one cases of schizophrenia. But a recent multiuniversity study of the families involved ruled out at least one gene mutation thought to be the culprit.

While studies do confirm evidence of brain abnormalities in schizophrenic patients, the exact way schizophrenia is passed on to children remains a mystery. First-degree relatives (parents, siblings, and children) of people with the illness have a 10 percent chance of getting this illness, compared to 1 percent for the overall population.

mitter) passed from generation to generation on her family tree? Her family has not been studied in this way, so there is no medical evidence to prove this assumption. However, it is a provocative and valid theory. Look at the problems in her family related to low serotonin levels:

Alcoholism

Eating disorders/obesity

Aggression (domestic physical abuse)

Obsessive sexual behavior (sexual abuse)

Unspecified mental illness

There is also the possibility of abnormally high serotonin levels in Sarah's family—at least two recorded cases of autism. It could be argued that uneven chemical levels run in families, whether they be too high or too low.

The high rate of alcohol and nicotine addiction in Sarah's family also suggests low levels of dopamine, with Sarah's relatives struggling to stimulate suppressed pleasure centers in the brain. Most of the problems of Sarah's family are treatable—either with medicine, psychiatry, or psychotherapy. But because behavior patterns must be identified before they can be treated, her family has lived over the years in a prison of ignorance, a sort of multigenerational behavioral purgatory.

Are these behavior patterns of conduct truly biological and genetic, or are they simply learned in childhood as youngsters mimic their parents' flawed approaches to life? Either way, Sarah's first step toward emotional recovery was making her genogram, because it forced her to find labels for the dangerous behavior of her relatives—and to trace the emergent patterns.

Next: It's your turn to begin the illuminating journey into an unexplored territory of your family pedigree—Your Own Genogram.

IS SUICIDE AN INHERITED TRAGEDY?

A new study says one out of every four people who attempts suicide has a family member who's also tried to commit suicide.

The study, sponsored by the National Institute of Mental Health, looked at 2,300 residents of Los Angeles. The study revealed that mental illness can create clusters of suicide attempts in families. Not surprisingly, the study also showed that the mental disorder of a parent (which may or may not result in suicide) can contribute to a person's sense of social isolation, and put one at higher risk for suicide.

The chief investigator of the study, Dr. Susan Sorenson, says future research will focus on how the family responds to suicide attempts.

There is no implication here that there is a suicide "gene." But the study does show why it is important to look at behavioral patterns in your family, and how your genogram can help you understand how your family has traditionally reacted to crises. Certainly in the case of suicide, such a desperate act is not inevitable simply because it has happened in your family before. But your family history is a powerful warning signal that everyone in your family needs to focus on recognizing symptoms of depression and developing strong coping skills.

YOUR OWN GENOGRAM
WORKBOOK

1. DETERMINE YOUR PAINPOINTS. What would you like to change or understand better about yourself? (For Samuel, his painpoints were "Anger," "Intolerance," and "Lack of Self-Acceptance.") List your top three.

"PAINPOINTS"

A re there aspects about yourself you would like to understand better or change? These painpoints should be the focus of your genogram.

The following is a list of descriptive feelings that you might have about yourself. These personality features can help put your emotions into words for your genogram. Or you may use your own descriptions or feelings. Remember that in Samuel's genogram, he chose the painpoints "Anger," "Intolerance," and "Lack of Self-Acceptance."

Anger *("I feel angry often, and sometimes I don't even know what I'm angry about.")*

Dishonesty *("I don't know why I do dishonest things.")*

Tyrant *("My father always had to have his way, or we would be severely punished.")*

Noncommunicative *("I find it so hard to communicate my feelings.")*

Possessive *("My wife says I'm too possessive.")*

Controlling *("My husband says I'm a control freak . . . I guess he's right, but that's just the way I am.")*

Can't say no *("I volunteered for another school project, but I don't really have the time.")*

Intolerant *("I just can't stand that type of person—and I refuse to work with anyone like that.")*

Feel unloved *("It doesn't matter what I do, my parents won't ever really love me.")*

Bad eating habits *("If I just had more willpower I would look and feel better. Sometimes I hate myself for the way I eat.")*

Obsessive *("I wish I could lighten up about housework, but it drives me crazy when anything is out of place, and I have to clean it up immediately. It seems that all I do is housework.")*

Fear *("I'd really like to change careers, but I'm afraid I would fail at something new.")*

Antisocial *("My brother always wants me to go out with his pals, but the thought just makes me too uncomfortable.")*

Hostile *("I really hate my boss, and if it weren't against the law I'd bash his head in.")*

"PAINPOINTS" (cont'd.)

Hurtful ("I know I promised not to tell my friend's secret to anyone, but I only told one person I thought I could trust. Why did I do that, anyway?")

Violent ("Next time I will try to control my temper better, but she makes me so angry that sometimes I think she's asking for it.")

Sexually Overactive ("I'm not sure why I end up in bed with people so quickly, and then regret it.")

Ashamed ("I can't talk to anyone about this.")

Substance abuse ("Maybe I have a little bit of a problem, but I could stop anytime I want.")

Uninvolved ("Sometimes I seem so separate from everyone else, they just aren't interested in anything I like.")

Smothering ("My son tells me to leave him alone. Doesn't he know I want to be involved in his life because I only want the best for him?")

Unassertive ("I am so angry I was treated that way. Why didn't I say anything?")

Hate myself ("It doesn't matter what I do, I always seem to screw things up.")

Feel unaccepted ("My father never compliments me on my successes and hard work.")

Incompetent ("Everyone else is so much better than me at the office. I'm better off when I stay in the background.")

Compulsive ("I try to watch my weight, but I can't seem to stop eating, even after I'm full.")

Habitual gambler ("I suppose I should stop betting, but it's so much fun. In fact, I look forward to it more than anything else.")

Cowardly ("I really want to help my wife through her illness, but I'm not sure she really wants me there at the hospital very much.")

Immoral ("Everyone does it.")

Anxiety-ridden ("I would just like to have a peaceful feeling once—even for an hour.")

Strict ("My children know I am the boss of my house. Until they are grown, my rules of behavior are nonnegotiable.")

Physically abusive ("Sometimes all that works is a little physical discipline.")

Extremely shy ("I will cross the street to avoid having to say hello to people I know, or I will pretend I don't see them.")

This list can also be a guideline for describing others on your genogram.

2. CONSTRUCT A BASIC FAMILY TREE (on a large sheet of paper). Include spouse (or significant other) children, siblings and their spouses (include step- or half-siblings), parents, stepparents, and grandparents. Add aunts, uncles, and family acquaintances if they had a major impact on your immediate family. Use the block graph format.

3. ADD MAJOR LIFE EVENTS: births, deaths, marriages, separations, divorces, job changes, household moves, and anything else that comes to mind.

4. ADD MAJOR DISEASES, MENTAL ILLNESSES, EMOTIONAL ISSUES (and approximate date of onset). Worksheets begin on page 150.

Beginning Genogram: Block Graph

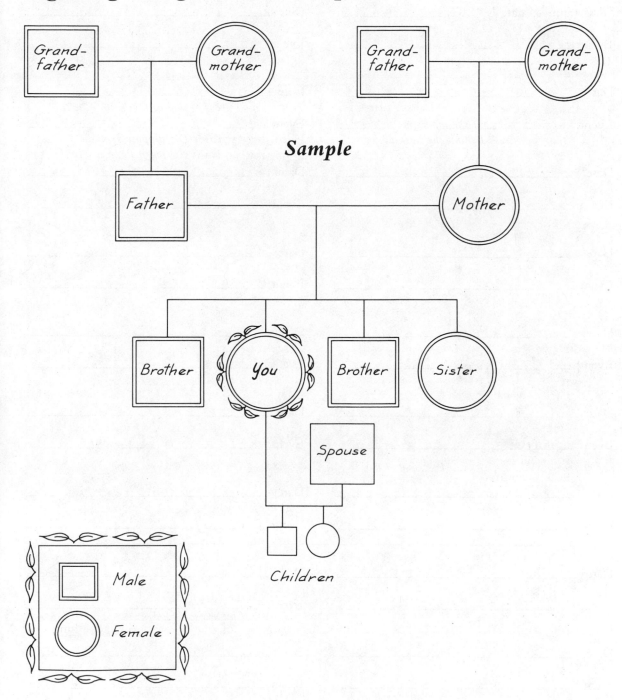

Sample

Grandfather · Grandmother · Grandfather · Grandmother

Father · Mother

Brother · You · Brother · Sister

Spouse

Children

Male

Female

LIFE EVENT WORKSHEET

Date: (approximate is O.K.) _____   Date: _____

Event: _____   Event: _____

Date: _____   Date: _____

Event: _____   Event: _____

Date: _____   Date: _____

Event: _____   Event: _____

Date: _____   Date: _____

Event: _____   Event: _____

Date: _____   Date: _____

Event: _____   Event: _____

Date: _____   Date: _____

Event: _____   Event: _____

Date: _____   Date: _____

Event: _____   Event: _____

Date: _____   Date: _____

Event: _____   Event: _____

Date: _____   Date: _____

Event: _____   Event: _____

Add more if necessary. Remember: Trust your instincts!

ILLNESS/EMOTIONS WORKSHEET

Date: _____

Illness/Emotional issue: _____

Onset: _____

Date: _____

Illness/Emotional issue: _____

Onset: _____

Date: _____

Illness/Emotional issue: _____

Onset: _____

Date: _____

Illness/Emotional issue: _____

Onset: _____

Date: _____

Illness/Emotional issue: _____

Onset: _____

Date: _____

Illness/Emotional issue: _____

Onset: _____

Date: _____

Illness/Emotional issue: _____

Onset: _____

Date: _____

Illness/Emotional issue: _____

Onset: _____

Date: _____

Illness/Emotional issue: _____

Onset: _____

Date: _____

Illness/Emotional issue: _____

Onset: _____

Date: _____

Illness/Emotional issue: _____

Onset: _____

Date: _____

Illness/Emotional issue: _____

Onset: _____

5. Note any missing information. Ask about more mysterious family members. Be curious. (Remember Samuel's discovery that helped explain his grandmother's anger at the world?)

6. Think about how separate people in the genogram relate to your painpoints. (In Samuel's case, he learned that anger, one of his painpoints, was a predominant personality feature of several people in his family.)

7. Describe significant relationships among members of your immediate family. To do this, draw lines between people's names on the genogram using these codes:

- CLOSE: Intimate, mutually supportive relationship that doesn't sacrifice appreciation of individual differences. DRAW THIS LINE: _____

- FUSED (OVERLY CLOSE): Inhibiting expression of individual thoughts and feelings (some people might describe this as "smothering").
  DRAW THIS LINE: ================

- DISTANT: Not much contact or conflict.
  DRAW THIS LINE: _ _ _ _ _ _ _ _ _ _

- CONFLICTUAL: Not intimate; argumentative.
  DRAW THIS LINE: \/\/\/\/\/\

- FUSED AND CONFLICTUAL: Neither one knows how to function individually or how to respect the need of the other to do so.
  DRAW THIS LINE: ⋈⋈⋈⋈⋈

- CUT OFF: Not talking, not tolerating.
  DRAW THIS LINE: ⊢———⊣ ⊢———⊣

Do not agonize over these terms. Trust your instincts, and use the descriptions that best fit.

8. LOOK AT THE COMPLETE GENOGRAM. WHICH EVENTS, PEOPLE, OR RELATIONSHIPS SEEM ESPECIALLY RELEVANT TO ONE OR MORE OF YOUR PAINPOINTS? To help you do this, ask one or more of the following questions:

A. What was it like to be in your important triangles?
B. What was it like to be in a triangle with your parents?
C. Which individuals have life experiences that seem related to your painpoints? Are any of these people in a triangle with you?

9. NOW ASK SIMILAR QUESTIONS FROM YOUR PARENTS' PERSPECTIVES:

A. What was it like for my mother to be in a triangle with my father and me?
B. What was it like for my mother to be in her family?
C. What was it like for my father to be in a triangle with my mother and me?
D. What was it like for my father to be in his family?

Add notes on other relatives if you believe their perspectives are important. For example, Samuel could have observed what it was like for his grandmother Dora to be in her family, after having lost her siblings to the Holocaust. Or Sarah could have asked her father's sisters what it was like to grow up with her father, who turned out to be a highly abusive adult.

10. Are you curious about how you relate to your spouse or significant other? You might want to do rough genograms of their lives as well. This can only be done successfully if:

A. Your partner is eager and willing.

B. You don't analyze them (most of us bristle when we receive uninvited analysis from a partner).

C. Don't tell your partner how to answer the genogram questions.

This can be a complicated undertaking and is at the core of some couples' counseling. If this is important to you, get the genograms started and possibly seek advice from a professional who is trained in family therapy. In the meantime, here are some questions you and your partner can explore after making a basic genogram:

1. What was it like for each of you to be in your father-mother-child triangle?

2. What other family triangles were each of you in? Describe them.

3. What was the best thing about being in your family?

4. What was the worst?

5. A question for men to ask: Do I remind you of your father? In what way? How am I different from your father?

6. A question for women to ask: Do I remind you of your mother? In what way? How am I different from your mother?

7. For both of you to answer: How did your parents/family resolve conflict? Give examples you remember.

8. How would you describe your mother's values? Your father's?

This is an especially good exercise to try before you marry. The genogram helps put into words and clarify your deepest values. If you find that your families resolved conflict quite differently, or that the two of you were raised with very different values, you might consider more extensive counseling. How your spouse related to his or her parents in the past can be an illuminating window to your future relationship.

11. Take your own genogram and extra notes to an "observer" to help you analyze it. This could be a close friend, spouse, or family therapist. You may need an objective eye. Tell your observer about your painpoints, then he or she can make any comments he or she believes are relevant. But you should start with these questions:

A. Do you see any patterns that relate to my painpoints?

B. Do you see any patterns of behavior in my family that relate to something other than my painpoints?

C. Do you see anything surprising? Something you didn't know about me or my family before?

12. FINAL STEP: ASK YOURSELF THESE QUESTIONS:

A. Am I following a pattern in my family?

B. Is there an unwritten rule that this is the way I am supposed to feel about, or perceive something?

C. What would happen *in my family* if I changed and managed my painpoints differently? What would each person say?

D. What's it like *for me* to try small changes in how I relate to key members of my family?

Remember there are no right or wrong answers in interpreting your genogram. You should come away with a better understanding of why you behave and feel the way you do. Congratulations and good luck!

This Genogram Workbook was created with the professional assistance of behavioral scientist Larry Mauksch, M.Ed., of the Department of Medicine at the University of Washington Department of Family Medicine in Seattle. My sincere thanks to him.

Larry Mauksch and his colleague Richard Weinberg, Ph.D., of the University of South Florida and the Florida Mental Health Institute, write and teach on the use of genograms in family and marital therapy and in the workplace. Their work on genograms can be studied in their article "Examining Family-of-Origin Influences in Life at Work," *Journal of Marital and Family Therapy,* Vol. 17, No. 3, 233-242, July 1991.

V

RESOURCES

WHERE TO WRITE
FOR DEATH CERTIFICATES

Alabama
*Alabama Department of Public
  Health
P.O. Box 5625
Montgomery, AL 36103-5625
205-242-5033
205-242-5041
Records from:
January 1908 to present
Fees:
$5.00 each
$2.00 each additional copy
$5.00 for express service + Fed-
  eral Express charges
Personal check payable to Alabama
State Board of Health*

Alaska
*Bureau of Vital Statistics
P.O. Box 110675
Juneau, AL 99811-0675
907-465-3391/2
Records from:
1920, some from 1913
Fees:
$7.00 each
$10.00 extra for Visa or Master-
  card
Check or money payable to Bu-
  reau of Vital Statistics*

Arizona
*Arizona Department of Vital
  Records
P.O. Box 3887
Phoenix, AZ 85030
Records from:
late 1800s
Fees:
$5.00 each
Certified check or money order
  payable to Arizona Department
  of Vital Records*

Arkansas
*Vital Records
Department of Health
4815 West Markham
Slot 44
Little Rock, AR 72205
Records from:
1914
Fees:
$4.00 each
$1.00 each additional copy
Check or money order payable to
  Arkansas Department of Health
For Visa or Mastercard call 501-
  661-2726
(additional charges will apply)*

California
*Office of the State Registrar
304 S Street
P.O. Box 730241
Sacramento, CA 95814-0241
916-445-2684
800-858-5553 (FAX)
Records from:
1880s
Fees:
$8.00 each
$8.00 extra for each 10-year search
$5.00 extra for Visa or Mastercard
Check or money order payable to
  Office of State Registrar*

Colorado
*Colorado Department of Vital
  Records
4210 East Eleventh Avenue
Denver, CO 80220
303-331-4893
Records from:
1900
Fees:
$12.00 each*

*$6.00 each additional copy
Visa or Mastercard additional
  $5.00 (303-893-6026)
Check or money order payable to
  Colorado Department of Vital
  Records*

Connecticut
*State Health Department
150 Washington Street
Hartford, CT 06106
203-722-6700
203-722-6701
Records from:
1897 for Connecticut
1852 for Hartford
Fees:
$5.00 each
Check or money order payable to
  City of Hartford*

Delaware
*Department of Vital Statistics
P.O. Box 637
Dover, DE 19903
302-739-4721
Records from:
1930
Fees:
$5.00 each
$3.00 each additional copy
Check or money order payable to
  Delaware Department of Vital
  Statistics*

**District of Columbia
  (Washington, D.C.)**
*Vital Records
425 I Street NW
3rd Floor
Washington, D.C. 20001
202-727-5314*

Records from:
 1874 to present
Fees:
 $8.00 each
 Check or money order payable to
  D. C. Treasurer

For Earlier Records:
 Division of Historic and Cultural
  Affairs
 Hall of Records
 Dover, DE 19901
 302-739-5318
Records from:
 Late 1600s to 1929
Fees:
 $5.00 each
 Check or money order payable to
  Delaware Division of Historic
  and Cultural Affairs

Florida
 Office of Vital Statistics
 P.O. Box 210
 Jacksonville, FL 32321
 904-359-6902
Records from:
 1917; some records as far back as
  1865
Fees:
 $5.00 each
 $4.00 each additional copy
 $2.00 each year for search
 Check or money order payable to
  Office of Vital Statistics

Georgia
 Vital Records Unit
 #217-H
 47 Trinity Avenue SW
 Atlanta, GA 30334
 404-656-4900
 404-656-7456
Records from:
 1919
Fees:
 $3.00 each
 $1.00 each additional copy
 Check or money order payable to
  Vital Records Service

Hawaii
 Vital Records Section
 State Department of Health

P.O. Box 3378
 Honolulu, HI 96801
 808-586-4533
 808-586-4539
Records from:
 1896; some districts as far back as
  1865 (mainly Honolulu)
Fees:
 $2.00 each
 Check or money order payable to
  State Department of Health

Idaho
 Department of Vital Statistics
 State House
 Boise, ID 83720
 208-334-5988
Records from:
 July 1911
Fees:
 $8.00 each
 Check or money order payable to
  Department of Vital Statistics

Illinois
 Division of Vital Records
 605 West Jefferson Street
 Springfield, IL 62702-5097
 217-782-6553
Records from:
 January 1916, prior in some counties
Fees:
 $15.00 each certified copy
 $10.00 each uncertified copy
 $2.00 each additional copy
 Check or money order payable to
  Illinois Department of Health

Indiana
 Indiana State Department of
  Health
 Vital Records
 1330 West Michigan Street
 Indianapolis, IN 46206
 317-633-0274
Records from:
 1900
Fees:
 $4.00 each
 $1.00 each additional copy
 Check or money order payable to
  Indiana State Department of
  Health

Iowa
 Iowa Department of Health
 Vital Records Division
 321 East 12th Street
 Lucas Building
 Des Moines, IA 50319
 515-281-4944
Records from:
 1880
Fees:
 $6.00 each
 $6.00 for each year searched
 Check or money order payable to
  Iowa Department of Health

Kansas
 Office of Vital Statistics
 900 South West Jackson
 Topeka, KS 66612-1290
 913-296-1400
Records from:
 1911; counties go back further
Fees:
 $7.00 each
 $4.00 each additional copy
 Check or money order payable to
  Office of Vital Statistics

Kentucky
 Cabinet for Human Resources
 Vital Statistics Division
 275 East Main Street
 Frankfort, KY 40621
 502-564-4212
Records from:
 1911. Four cities go further back:
 Louisville   1866–1911
 Lexington   1898–1911
 Covington   1880–1911
 Newport   1884–1911
Fees:
 $5.00 each
 Check or money order payable to
  Kentucky State Treasurer

Louisiana
 Vital Records Registry
 P.O. Box 60630
 New Orleans, LA 70160
 504-568-5152
 504-568-5391 (FAX)
Records from:
 Less than fifty years old

Fees:
  $5.00 each
  *Check or money order payable to
    Vital Records Registry. $15.00
    extra for Federal Express*

For Earlier Records:
  *Louisiana State Archives
  P.O. Box 94125
  Baton Rouge, LA 70804
  504-922-1206*
Records from:
  fifty or more years old
Fees:
  $5.00 each
  *Check or money order payable to
    Louisiana State Archives.
    $15.00 extra for Federal Express*

Maine
  *Department of Vital Records
  State House Station II
  Augusta, ME 04333
  207-289-3184*
Records from:
  1923
Fees:
  $4.00 each
  *Check or money order to
    Treasurer, State of Maine
  Visa or Mastercard $5.00 extra
    (207-289-3181)*

For Earlier Records:
  *Maine State Archives
  Statehouse Station 84
  Augusta ME 04333-0084
  207-289-5790*
Records from:
  Prior to 1923

Maryland
  *Division of Vital Records
  P.O. Box 68760
  Baltimore, MD 21215
  800-832-3277
  410-764-3038*
Records from:
  1969
Fees:
  $4.00 each
  *Check or money order payable to
    Division of Vital Records*

For Earlier Records:
  *State Archives
  305 Rowe Boulevard
  Annapolis, MD 21401
  410-974-3914*
Records from:
  *1874–1982 for city of Baltimore
  1875–1982 for county
  1898–1969 state*
Fees:
  $4.00 each
  *Check or money order payable to
    Maryland State Archives*

Massachusetts
  *Registrar of Vital Records
  150 Tremont
  Boston, MA 02111
  617-727-0036*
Records from:
  1900
Fees:
  $6.00 each
  *Check or money order payable to
    Commonwealth of Massachusetts*

For Earlier Records:
  *Massachusetts State Archives at
    Columbia Point
  220 Morrissey Boulevard
  Boston, MA 02125-3314*
Records from:
  Prior to 1900

Michigan
  *Michigan Department of Health
  Office of State Registrar
  P.O. Box 30195
  Lansing, MI 48909
  517-335-8656*
Records from:
  1867
Fees:
  $10.00 each
  $3.00 each additional copy
  *Check or money order payable to
    State of Michigan*

Minnesota
  *Minnesota Department of Health
  717 Delaware Street SE
  Minneapolis, MN 55440
  RE: Death Certificate
  612-623-5121*

Records from:
  *1908. Inquiries for years prior
    1908 should be made to the indi-
    vidual county*
Fees:
  $8.00 each
  $2.00 each additional copy
  *Check or money order payable to
    the Minnesota Department of
    Health*

Mississippi
  *Mississippi State Board of Health
  P.O. Box 1700
  Jackson, MS 39215
  RE: Death Certificate
  601-960-7981*
Records from:
  *1912 (for certified copy). No
    death certificates prior to 1912
    but cemetery, genealogical, and
    will records can be obtained from:
  Library, Mississippi Department
    of Archives & History
  P.O. Box 571
  Jackson, MS 39205
  $10.00 research fee for mail request*
Fees:
  $10.00 each
  $2.00 each additional copy
  *Check or money order payable to
    Mississippi State Board of
    Health*

Missouri
  *Missouri Department of Health
  Bureau of Vital Records
  P.O. Box 570
  Jefferson City, MO 65102-0570
  314-751-6400*
Records from:
  1910
Fees:
  $5.00 each
  *Check or money order payable to
    Missouri Department of Health*

Montana
  *Vital Records
  Montana Department of Health
  1400 Broadway
  Helena, MT 59620
  406-444-2614*

Records from:
  1920s; some records go back to
    1860
Fees:
  $10.00 each
  $10.00 for each five-year search
  Check or money order payable to
    Montana Department of Health

Nebraska
  Bureau of Vital Records
  State Department of Health
  P.O. Box 95007
  Lincoln, NE 68509-5007
  402-471-2871
Records from:
  1904
Fees:
  $5.00 each
  Check or money order payable to
    Bureau of Vital Records

Nevada
  Vital Statistics
  505 East King Street
  Carson City, NV 89710
  702-687-4480
Records from:
  1911; inquiries for years prior to
    1911 should be made to the indi-
    vidual county
Fees:
  $8.00 each
  Check or money order payable to
    Vital Statistics

New Hampshire
  Vital Records
  6 Hazen Drive
  Concord, NH 03301-6527
  603-271-4654
Records from:
  1640
Fees:
  $10.00 each
  Check or money order to Treasurer
    State of New Hampshire. $6.00
    extra charge for Visa or Master-
    card (603-271-4650)

New Jersey
  Bureau of Vital Statistics
  CN-370
  Trenton, NJ 08625
  609-292-4087

Records from:
  1878
Fees:
  $4.00 each
  $2.00 each additional copy
  $1.00 per year for search
  Check or money order payable to
    Bureau of Vital Statistics. $5.00
    extra for Visa or Mastercard.
    Exact information is needed
    (609-633-2860)

New Mexico
  Vital Records
  P.O. 26110
  Sante Fe, NM 87502
  505-827-2338
  505-827-0121
Records from:
  1920
Fees:
  $5.00 each
  Check or money order payable to
    New Mexico Vital Records

New York City
  Bureau of Vital Records
  New York City Department of
    Health
  125 Worth Street
  New York, NY 10013
  212-788-4520-25
Records from:
  1898
Fees:
  $15.00 each
  $3.00 for each year searched
  Certified check or money order
    payable to Bureau of Vital
    Records

For Earlier Records:
New York City
  Municipal Archives
  31 Chambers Street, #103
  New York, NY 10007
  212-566-5292
Records from:
  1795 for Manhattan
  1847 for Brooklyn
  1898 for Bronx
  1880 for Queens
  1880 for Richmond
Fees:
  $15.00 each

  $3.00 for each year searched
  Certified check or money order
    payable to Bureau of Vital
    Records

New York State
  New York State Department of
    Health
  Office of Vital Records
  Empire State Plaza
  Albany, NY 12237
  518-474-3077
Records from:
  1880; for years prior to 1880 con-
    tact local registrar, city, or county
Fees:
  $15.00 each
  Check or money order payable to
    New York State Department of
    Health

North Carolina
  Vital Records
  P.O. Box 29537
  Raleigh, NC 27626
  919-733-3526
Records from:
  1930
Fees:
  $10.00 each
  $5.00 each additional copy
  Check or money order payable to
    Vital Records

For Earlier Records:
  History and Archives
  109 East Jones
  Raleigh, NC 27602
  919-733-3526
Records from:
  1913
Fees:
  $10.00 each
  $5.00 each additional copy
  Check or money order payable to
    History and Archives

North Dakota
  Vital Records
  Capitol Building
  600 East Boulevard
  Bismarck, ND 58505
  701-224-2360

Records from:
1893
Fees:
$5.00 each
$2.00 each additional copy
Check or money order payable to
Vital Records

Ohio

Bureau of Vital Statistics
Ohio Department of Health
P.O. Box 15098
Columbus, OH 43215-0098
614-466-2531
Records from:
January 1937
Fees:
$7.00 each
Check or money order payable to
State Treasurer of Ohio

For Earlier Records:
Ohio Historic Society
1985 Belma Street
Columbus, OH 43211
614-297-2300
Records from:
1908; some individual county
records go back further
Fees:
$7.00 each
Check or money order payable to
Ohio Historic Society

Oklahoma

Vital Records
State Department of Health
P.O. Box 53551
Oklahoma City, OK 73152
405-271-4040
Records from:
1908; records were not required
until 1940
Fees:
$5.00 each
$5.00 search fee
Check or money order payable to
State Department of Health

Special:
Other information available at:
State Historical Society
2100 North Lincoln
Oklahoma City, OK 73105
405-521-2491

Oregon

Vital Records
P.O. Box 14050
Portland, OR 97214
503-731-4095
503-731-4108
Records from:
1903
Fees:
$13.00 each
Check or money order payable to
Oregon Health Division

For Earlier Records:
Oregon State Archives
1005 Broadway North East
Salem, OR 97310
503-378-4241
Records from:
1862
Fees:
$13.00 each
Check or money order payable to
Oregon Health Division

Pennsylvania

Vital Records
P.O. Box 1528
New Castle, PA 16103
412-656-3100
Records from:
1906; individual counties have
records prior to 1906; some go as
far back as 1870
Fees:
$3.00 each
Check or money order payable to
Vital Records; self-addressed
stamped envelope required

Rhode Island

State of Rhode Island
Department of Health
Cannon Building, Room 101
3 Capitol Hill
Providence, RI 02908-5097
401-277-2812
Records from:
1853; counties have records prior
to 1853
Fees:
$10.00 each
$5.00 each additional copy

Check or money order payable to
General Treasurer State of
Rhode Island

South Carolina

Office of Vital Records
2600 Bull Street
Columbia, SC 29201
803-734-4830
Records from:
January 1915
Fees:
$8.00 each
$3.00 each additional copy
Check or money order payable to
DHEC

For Earlier Records:
Department of Archives
P.O. Box 11669
1430 Senate Street
Columbia, SC 29211
803-734-8596
Records from:
Years before 1915
Fees:
$8.00 each
$3.00 each additional copy
Check or money order payable to
DHEC

South Dakota

Department of Health
c/o Vital Records
445 East Castle
Pierre, SD 57501-3185
605-773-3355
605-733-4961
Records from:
July 1905
Fees:
$5.00 each
Check or money order payable to
South Dakota Department of
Health

Tennessee

Tennessee Department of Vital
Records
C-3-324 Cordell Hull Building
Nashville, TN 37247-0350
615-741-1763
Records from:
1942

Fees:
 $5.00 each
 Check or money order payable to
 Tennessee Department of Vital
 Records

For Earlier Records:
 State Library and Archives
 403 7th Avenue North
 Nashville, TN 37243-0312
 615-741-2764
 Records from:
 1908–1912 and 1914–1942

Texas
 Bureau of Vital Statistics
 1100 West 49th Street
 Austin, TX 78756-3191
 512-458-7111
 Records from:
 1903
 Fees:
 $9.00 each
 $3.00 each additional copy
 Check or money order payable to
 Vital Records

Utah
 Bureau of Vital Records
 P.O. Box 16700
 Salt Lake City, UT 84116-0700
 801-538-6186
 801-538-6380
 Records from:
 1905; some counties prior to that
 Fees:
 $9.00 each
 $5.00 each additional copy
 Check or money order payable to
 Bureau of Vital Records

Vermont
 Vital Records
 Vermont Department of Health
 P.O. Box 70
 Burlington, VT 05402
 802-863-7275
 Records from:
 1981 to present
 Fees:
 $5.00 each
 Check or money order payable to
 Division of Vital Records, Ver-
 mont Department of Health

For Earlier Records:
 Public Records Division
 U.S. Route 7-Middlesex
 133 State Street
 Montpelier, VT 05633-7601
 802-828-3286
 Records from:
 1700s
 Fees:
 $5.00 each
 Check or money order payable to
 Division of Vital Records,
 Vermont Department of Health

Virginia
 Division of Vital Records
 P.O. Box 1000
 Richmond VA 23208–1000
 804-786-6228
 Records from:
 1853–1896 and 1912 to present.
 From 1896 to 1912 there are no
 records (some larger cities have
 them)
 Fees:
 $5.00 each
 Check or money order payable to
 Virginia Division of Vital
 Records

Washington
 Center for Health Statistics
 P.O. 9709
 Olympia, WA 98504
 206-753-5936
 Records from:
 July 1907; counties prior
 Fees:
 $11.00 each
 Check or money order payable to
 Center for Health Statistics

West Virginia
 Vital Records Registration Office
 Capital Complex
 Building 3, Room 516
 Charleston, WV 25305
 304-348-2931
 Records from:
 1919; might be able to obtain ear-
 lier records from state archives
 Fees:
 $5.00 each
 Check or money order payable to
 Vital Records Registration Office

Wisconsin
 Vital Records
 P.O. Box 309
 Madison WI 53701
 608-266-1372
 Records from:
 1830s in some counties
 Fees:
 $7.00 each
 $2.00 each additional copy
 $7.00 for each five-year search
 Check or money order payable to
 Vital Records

Wyoming
 Vital Records
 Hathaway Building
 Cheyenne, WY 82002
 307-777-7591
 Records from:
 1908
 Fees:
 $6.00 each
 Check or money order payable to
 Vital Records

Territories

GUAM:
 Department of Health/Social
 Service
 P.O. Box 2816
 Guam 96910
 Send $1.00 money order

PUERTO RICO:
 Demographic Registry
 P.O. Box 11854
 San Juan, Puerto Rico 00910
 Send $2.00 money order and a
 photocopy of your identification
 (drivers license preferred

U.S. VIRGIN ISLANDS:
 St. Thomas:
 Department of Health
 Vital Statistics
 Old Municipal Hospital
 St. Thomas, Virgin Islands 00802

St. Croix:
Department of Health/Vital
  Statistics
Charles Harrold Memorial
  Hospital
Christiansted
St. Croix, Virgin Islands 00820

*Death certificate copies will cost
$10 but do not send it in your
first letter. You will be sent a
form to fill out and mail with the
fee.
For other islands, contact the Department of Public Health of that
island. Dial directory assistance
(1/809/555-1212) for the number.*

Special Resources for Common Racial, Cultural, and Ethnic Groups

African-American:

The book and miniseries Roots inspired Americans of all colors to research their ancestry. But Africans brought to this country as slaves were usually not allowed to use their birth name and were instead given an American first name with no surname. So blacks in this country have special difficulties finding information about their ancestors.

Oddly enough, the same disrespect often shown for the importance and independence of slave families during those years has also left some genealogical clues. The Source, A Guidebook of American Genealogy (Ancestry Publishing) cites a study that might surprise you: that 75 percent of American blacks have at least one white ancestor. That increases the likelihood that some records were kept.

Also, by 1860, one of eight slaves were already freed and began to take on last names, making families more traceable even before the Civil War.

To identify a slave ancestor, your best lead is to identify the plantation and focus on the records of that family. As crude as it sounds, slave purchases and sales were often recorded as business transactions.

For Help:
Freedman's Bureau Field Office
  Records
The National Archives
(See pages 165–66 for address of
  closest National Archives branch)

The Registry of Black American
  Ancestry
The Genealogical Society of Utah
35 N.W. Temple Street
Salt Lake City, UT 84150
801-240-2331

Beginning an African-American
  Genealogical Pursuit (1985), by
  Jean Sampson Scott. Send $5.00
  to Professor Osborne E. Scott (her
  husband), 323 Egmont Avenue.
  Mt. Vernon, NY 10553

African-American Cultural Museum
701 Arch Street
Philadelphia, PA 19106
215-574-0380

Hispanic/Spanish:

Here is a culture filled with family Bibles, which can be one of the best resources in the Christian world for very special, detailed family histories. In the same spirit of family pride, Catholic institutions have also kept good records over the years. Start with your local diocese for referrals to local historical and genealogical societies.

But record-keeping in America's Southwest was not always done out of family pride. The Spanish government gave away land to encourage settlements and to convert Native American Indians to Christianity.

Because most of the early Spanish pioneers settled in Texas, New Mexico, California, and Arizona, those states would be good places to search for your family name. (See the list of regional offices of the National Archives on pages 165–66.)

For Help:
There are some records that date as far back as 1721 that were kept by the Catholic Church Missions in Texas. You can check with the

Archdiocese of San Antonio
2718 West Woodlawn
San Antonio, TX 78228
512-734-2620

Contact the Spanish-language newspaper that best reports on your home of origin. Again, you might get a referral to a useful historical society *that can help you search in Mexico, Spain, even Puerto Rico.*

Asian-American:

There are about four million Americans of Asian descent, most commonly coming from China, Japan, Korea, The Philippines, and Southeast Asia. Each culture has its own birth and burial rituals, spiritual mood, and approach to record-keeping. The Chinese were essentially the first to arrive, but most of this immigration is fairly recent.

First, try the traditional sources: old family records, documents, and conversations with elderly relatives to try and identify the geographical origin of the family and the port of entry, which will most probably be on the West Coast or in Hawaii.

For Help:
Contact the offices of the Asian-language newspapers found in larger cities. Staffers can lead you to historians and genealogists who specialize in your family's original home.

Try the records of the Immigration and Naturalization Service. There are more than fifty INS offices around the country, and records there might help you identify the port of entry for certain family names.

Native Americans:

Ironically, it might be those whose ancestors have been in America the longest who have the toughest time building a family tree. Many Native Americans were forced to leave their lands and were slaughtered or died by the thousands from diseases introduced by white settlers, most notably smallpox. So they were often wandering civilizations that had little motivation for lugging around family records, despite great pride in family life.

Yet Native American culture and lore is rich and deep, and simple memories from elder citizens might be a superb source for information. And there are actually census records for some tribes, especially what the government noted as the Five Civilized Tribes—the Cherokee, Chickasaw, Choctaw, Creek, and Seminole.

For Help:
The National Archives has the largest collection of Native American census records, including individual tribal rolls that predate 1900, much of it recorded by the Bureau of Indian Affairs.
(See pages 165–66 for locations of Archive offices)

The second largest collection of Native American or "Indian" documents is at the Indiana Archives of Oklahoma. It is maintained by the Oklahoma Historical Society. The entire state was once Indian territory, and the collection of documents is impressive.

Indiana Archives
Oklahoma Historical Society
2100 North Lincoln Boulevard
Oklahoma City, OK 73105
405-521-2491

Jewish Family Records:

The uprooting of so many Jews during the Holocaust has naturally complicated the search for Jewish ancestry overseas. Even so, the library of the Genealogical Society of Utah has microfilm of genealogical records of some West German towns and villages. Soon, East German records may be made available to Americans.

To locate the ancestral home, consulting family papers and older members of the family are your best resources.

For research on ancestors in this country, records surrounding religious ceremonies can be your best bets:

1. American synagogue records
2. Religious school registries
3. Birth and circumcision records
4. Bar and bat mitzvah records
5. Death and cemetery documents

For Help:
The Genealogical Society of Utah
32 N.W. Temple Street
Salt Lake City, UT 84150
801-240-2331

Ask a local rabbi. What better source to get a referral to a local Jewish historical society?

RESOURCES

Books:

The Source—A Guidebook of American Genealogy
Edited by Arlene Eakle and Johni Cerny
Ancestry Publishing
This is the best reference book for genealogy, although it is huge and somewhat cumbersome. If you are serious, this will tell you everything you need to know, including excellent research sources for different minority and ethnic cultures.

The Handy Book for Genealogists
The Everton Publishers, Inc.
P.O. Box 368
Logan, UT 84321
This book will give you state-by-state information and help you locate ancestors by identifying their genealogical roots. Then you can proceed to search local cemeteries, church records, libraries, etc.

Do People Grow on Family Trees?
by Ira Wolfman
Workman Publishing
For children or even beginning adults, it concentrates on immigrants to Ellis Island and is a delight to read, with wonderful photos.

Unpuzzling Your Past
by Emily Anne Croom
Betterway Publications
Great copies of all the genealogical forms you might need.

Genetic Nutrition: Designing a Diet Based on Your Family Medical History
by Artemis Simopoulos, Victor Herbert, and Beverly Jacobson
Macmillan Publishing
This book discusses the critical role your genetic make-up plays in your susceptibility to disease and offers detailed information on what to eat—and what to avoid—if you have a family history of cancer, diabetes, heart disease, food allergies, obesity, or other conditions in which heredity plays a part.

Using The National Archives to Get Just About Any Information You Need

Genealogical information
Census records
Records about Native Americans
Land records
Naturalization records
Immigration passenger lists
Passport applications
Personnel records
Claims for pensions and bounty land
Military service records
Contact any of the regional offices of The National Archives. Staffers will help you locate information on ancestors and missing relatives.

The National Archives
Main Branch
Eighth Street and Pennsylvania Avenue, NW
Washington, D.C. 20536

NEW ENGLAND REGION
380 Trapelo Road
Waltham, MA 02154
617-647-8100
Covers Connecticut, Maine, Massachusetts, New Hampshire, Rhode Island, and Vermont.

NORTHEAST REGION
201 Varick Street
New York, NY
10014-4811
212-337-1300
Covers New Jersey, New York, Puerto Rico, and the Virgin Islands.

MID-ATLANTIC REGION
Ninth and Market Streets, Room 1350
Philadelphia, PA 19107
215-597-3000
Covers Delaware, Maryland, Pennsylvania, Virginia, and West Virginia.

SOUTHEAST REGION
1557 St. Joseph Avenue
East Point, GA 30344
404-763-7477
Covers Alabama, Georgia, Florida, Kentucky, Mississippi, North Carolina, South Carolina, and Tennessee.

GREAT LAKES REGION
7358 South Pulaski Road
Chicago, IL 60629
312-581-7816
Covers Illinois, Indiana, Michigan, Minnesota, Ohio, and Wisconsin.

CENTRAL PLAINS REGION
2312 East Bannister Road
Kansas City, MO 64131
816-926-6272
Covers Iowa, Kansas, Missouri,
and Nebraska.

SOUTHWEST REGION
501 West Felix Street (building
address)
P.O. Box 6216 (mailing address)
Fort Worth, TX 76115
817-334-5525
Covers Arkansas, Louisiana, New
Mexico, Oklahoma, and Texas.

ROCKY MOUNTAIN REGION
Building 48, Denver Federal
Center
Denver, CO 80225-0307
303-236-0817
Covers Colorado, Montana, North
Dakota, South Dakota, Utah, and
Wyoming.

PACIFIC SOUTHWEST RE-
GION
24000 Avila Road (building ad-
dress)
P.O. Box 6719 (mailing address)
Laguna Niguel, CA 92607-6719
714-643-4241
Covers Arizona, the Southern
California counties of Imperial,
Inyo, Kern, Los Angeles, Orange,
Riverside, San Bernadino, San
Diego, San Luis Obisbo, Santa
Barbara, Ventura, and Nevada's
Clark County.

PACIFIC SIERRA REGION
1000 Commodore Drive
San Bruno, CA 94066
415-876-9009
Covers Hawaii, Nevada (except
Clark County), northern California, and the Pacific Ocean area.

PACIFIC NORTHWEST RE-
GION
6125 Sand Point Way
Seattle, WA 98115
206-526-6507

Covers Alaska, Idaho, Oregon,
and Washington.

ALASKA REGION
654 West Third Avenue
Anchorage, AK 99501
907-271-2441
Alaska only.

Family Medical History

General Hereditary Diseases:

The Hereditary Disease Foundation
1427 7th Street, Suite 2
Santa Monica, CA 90401
213-458-4183
(Uses Huntington's chorea as model
to study family-related disorders.)

Hereditary Heart Disease:

• The American Heart Association
7320 Greenville Avenue
Dallas, TX 75231
214-373-6300
(For general information.)

• University of Utah Cardiovascular
Genetics Research Clinic410
Chipeta Way
• Research Park
Salt Lake City, UT 84108
(Dr. Roger Williams and his col-
leagues have been heading an
ongoing Family Tree Screening
Project with one of the best fam-
ily tree questionnaires I have ever
seen. Send for it!)

An excellent book:
If It Runs in Your Family: Heart
Disease
By Charles Klieman, M.D.,
and Scott Osborne
Bantam Books

Genograms

Genograms in Family Assessment
By Monica McGoldrick and Randy
Gerson
W.W. Norton
This is primarily a textbook for
therapists-in-training. It is an interesting read for those who want
to know more details about genograms.

Hereditary Cancers:

ALL CANCERS:
The Hereditary Cancer Institute
Creighton University School of
Medicine
California at 24th Streets
Omaha, NE
402-280-2942
This wonderful institution, headed
by Dr. Henry Lynch, offers free
cancer-risk information and genetic
counseling. You can request forms
that help you complete a medical
family tree.

The National Cancer Institute
Office of Cancer Communications
9000 Rockville Pike
Building 31, Room 10A24
Bethesda, MD 20014
National Hotline: 800-
4CANCER
The NCI gives free pamphlets and
referrals to certified local facilities.

American Cancer Society National
Office
1599 Clifton Road NE
Atlanta, GA 30329
National Hotline: 800-ACS-2345

Breast Cancer:
The National High-Risk Regis-
try/Strang Cancer Prevention
Center
428 East 72nd Street
New York, NY 10021
Free risk-monitoring if two close
relatives have been diagnosed with
breast cancer, or a mother, sister,

or daughter was diagnosed at a young age.

Ovarian Cancer:
Gilda Radner Familial Ovarian
Cancer Registry
Roswell Park Cancer Institute
Elm and Carlton Streets
Buffalo, NY 14260
Phone: 800-OVARIAN
Headed by Dr. Steven Piver, this registry has been keeping track of ovarian cancer families for more than a decade.

Genetic Counseling:

The National Society of Genetic
  Counselors
233 Canterbury Drive
Wallingford, PA 19086

This is a good place to start to receive information on the genetic counseling center nearest you.

Genealogy:

The Genealogical Society of Utah
(Church of Jesus Christ of Latter
  Day Saints)
35 N.W. Temple Street
Salt Lake City, UT 84150
801-240-2331
The Family History Library here is second to none. It has grown out of the Morman tradition of tracing family ancestry, although it covers just about every culture, ethnic group and national background. There are branches all over the country and the world. Call for the one nearest you.

Federation of Genealogical Societies
P.O. Box 220
Davenport, IA 52805
Write and ask them to send you the name of the genealogical society in your geographical area of interest. For greater specificity, you may want to give them the names and ethnic backgrounds of families you want to research.

Where to Write for Vital
  Records
A government booklet. To obtain a copy, write:
Superintendent of Documents
U.S. Government Printing Office
Washington, D.C. 20402